Beyond DESIRE

rediscovering health and wellness

Mark W. Hatcher, MD

iUniverse, Inc.
Bloomington

Beyond Desire
Rediscovering Health and Wellness

iUniverse books may be ordered through booksellers or by contacting:

iUniverse
1663 Liberty Drive
Bloomington, IN 47403
www.iuniverse.com
1-800-Authors (1-800-288-4677)

All photographs courtesy of Mike Donnelly(innerlighteditions.smugmug.com)

ISBN: 978-1-4620-4624-9 (sc)
ISBN: 978-1-4620-4625-6 (hc)
ISBN: 978-1-4620-4626-3 (e)

Printed in the United States of America

iUniverse rev. date: 08/31/2011

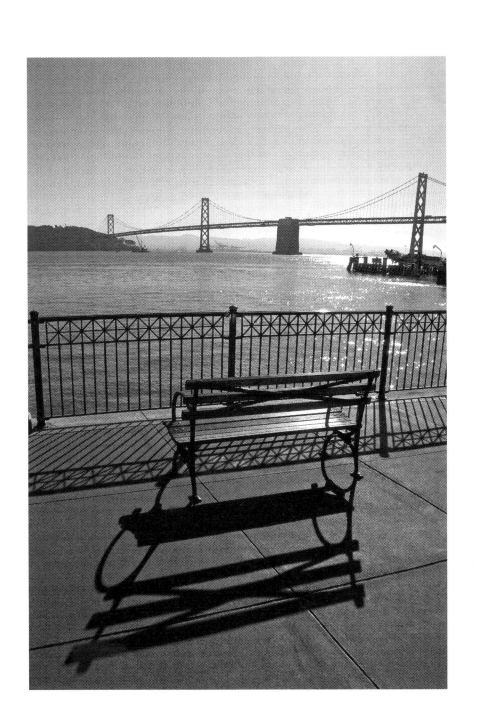

Contents

Though our outer nature is wasting away, our inner nature is being renewed every day. For this slight momentary affliction is preparing for us an eternal weight of glory beyond all comparison, because we look not to the things that are seen but to the things that are unseen.

Paul of Tarsus

All visible objects, man, are but as pasteboard masks. But in each event—in the living act, the undoubted deed—there, some unknown but still reasoning thing puts forth the moulding of its features from behind the unreasoning mask. If man will strike, strike through the mask!

Captain Ahab, *Moby Dick*

Introduction

Give me truths, for I am weary of the surfaces, and die of inanition.

R. W. Emerson

You are anxious and troubled about many things; only one thing is needful.

Jesus of Nazareth

On a cold winter morning in my busy urban emergency department I was given a moment of clarity. I could not help my patients.

Don't misunderstand me. I am an experienced emergency physician. I had an excellent liberal arts undergraduate education and then studied medicine at a well-respected medical school. Subsequently, I trained in my specialty of emergency medicine for three years, passed my specialty boards, and have been practicing now for fifteen years at a high-volume, hospital-based emergency department/trauma center. I adhere to the standards of practice that are accepted by my peers with regard to current diagnostics and therapeutics. In short, I know how to take care of acutely ill or injured people.

In the department on this morning were the following:

- a young business executive having chest pains, with normal stress-test imaging, cardiograms, radiographs, and blood testing

- a depressed middle-aged woman who had been taking antidepressant medication for years and now felt even more empty and hopeless and was suicidal

- an elderly female with progressive dementia who had become more confused and more difficult for the nursing home staff to manage

- an obese truck driver with chronic back pain who, despite several surgeries and pain management, was still experiencing debilitating pain

- an exhausted mother with her two children, all of whom had viral upper respiratory infections, who wanted to get some antibiotics

- a middle-aged divorcée who has been struggling with fibromyalgia for years and was in the department for the third time this month requesting pain relief

- an unemployed young man who just wanted to get high and had chest pain following the ingestion of narcotics and alcohol

- a divorced mother of four with persistent migraine headaches despite taking appropriate medicines as prescribed by her doctor

- a widowed, retired man with years of abdominal pain for which extensive testing had not found a cause

As I was sitting looking at their charts it became obvious to me that modern medicine had little to offer these people to heal their minds, bodies, and, least of all, their spirits. This insight occurred to a physician practicing medicine in the wealthiest nation with more resources at his disposal to help people and alleviate suffering than at any other time in the history of mankind. Yet, there I sat, helpless to heal these people in the midst of their pain. I prescribed medicines for them according to established practice patterns, made appropriate diagnostic assumptions, and moved on to the next onslaught of patients. However, now I was on a quest.

The questions can be summarized succinctly. Why are these people sick? What exactly is their disease? How can the modern practitioner of medicine assist the healing process? The prevailing philosophy of Western medicine is that of materialism. It is the accepted theory of medical teaching and practice. This doctrine teaches that the body is composed of organ systems, tissues, cells, and ultimately chemicals interacting in a precise and well-regulated dance that can be manipulated and controlled by an array of pharmaceuticals to encourage and/or cause healing.

Structural incompetency is the manifestation and hallmark of disease as symptoms of dysfunction become apparent. In severe cases of organ-system dysfunction a surgeon can intervene to remove or manipulate the diseased organ to affect the state of the disease. Other interventions can be utilized, such as the insertion of specialized catheters or imaging devices to alter disease processes.

The modern diagnostic disciplines of pathology and radiology accurately reveal the body's inner mechanisms. These analyses reveal disease states and structural abnormalities. In the course of my medical career, surgical techniques have been optimized, such as using endoscopy and minimally invasive interventions to diagnose and treat a wide array of disease states. Science can be used to find solutions for the problems that plague mankind. But I was faced with a department full of patients whose scientific evaluations revealed no abnormalities, yet still they were suffering. What was causing their symptoms?

The great success story of modern medicine is the proven use of pharmacologic and surgical therapies to treat the human body in crisis. This has done much to alleviate pain and suffering in the modern world. However, what happens when physicians do not find a body system in crisis? For this we have no answer. We do not want for a plethora of assumptions, however. We in the modern scientific community have posited a litany of theories on the causation of hypertension, atherosclerosis, cancer, mental health disorders, infections, dementia, and endocrine disease, to name a few.

Many of these theories have become entombed in our cultural thinking as fact, and physicians, hospitals, and the pharmaceutical industry have certainly profited handsomely from these assumptions. Without question many people have benefited from these advances. However, many more do not benefit, or have symptoms that seem to evade the omniscient eye of modern science. To whom could I turn to find answers when modern medical therapies were not helping?

It seemed clear that *materia medica* could not help. The mentors of my youth would turn to the halls of science for ultimate answers. Scientific investigation has proven to be inadequate in meeting the needs of many of my patients. Therefore, I have been led on a fascinating and enlightening journey to the wisdom of the sages and prophets of the ages, both modern and ancient. The central questions of life remain the same and cannot be answered by scientism. We are more than simply flesh. Our world is bathed in mystery. Perhaps our knowledge and information in this modern era is incomplete.

Accompany me on a journey to examine the assumptions upon which our modern world is founded. It is the claim of this author that much more is going on in the world and with our bodies than can be explained in whole or even in part through scientific inquiry or with the modern theories regarding human behavior.

Then hear what the world's great teachers have to say regarding our understanding of the self. It will be seen that the modern pursuits for pleasure, power, comfort, and security create inappropriate desires. These desires lead to imbalanced, unreleased energies that can result in disease states. We will explore the methods of healing that for centuries have been practiced by healers around the world to rebalance and release these energies. Finally, I will propose a strategy for health, bringing us to the realization that true healing does indeed lie beyond desire.

Let us begin this saga in the rooms of my busy ER. I invite the reader to come on rounds with me as my patients tell their stories— stories that are both individual and universal; symptoms of a culture in crisis.

Prologue: Lost in America

You're going the wrong way!

From the movie
Planes, Trains, and Automobiles

What is Truth?

Pontius Pilate

I have just started my night shift in a busy urban emergency department. It is 10:00 p.m. on a typical weekday night. Seven charts await me in the rack, each of which outlines the patient's chief complaint, a brief nurse's assessment, and an order sheet for my notes, treatments, and diagnostics. Two more sips of black coffee and off we go.

Robert M.

The forty-three-year-old confidently meets my gaze as I enter the examination room, and he calmly puts down his newspaper. Immediately he strikes me as a successful man of the business or legal world. Control is an integral part of his style. He is well-dressed and well-kempt. He is already attached to the technologic entrapments of the ER experience: blood pressure cuff, heart monitor, oxygen monitor, and call light (with radio and television switches). His wife sits next to him, distracted but concerned.

After returning from an important business trip earlier in the day, this evening he experienced chest pains while helping his wife put their three young children to bed for the night. The pains only lasted a few minutes, but there were three distinct episodes. He broke out in a sweat and also felt nauseous. Now the symptoms are gone. Upon further prompting he admits to having experienced similar episodes on this past week's trip, typically occurring during meetings. He has recently been sleeping poorly, and his diet has been consisting of a lot of fast foods. His alcohol and caffeine ingestion has been increasing in the past few months.

He admits to having occasional spells of heartburn, but this feels different. Cardiac risk factors include a strong family history (his father had a heart attack in his forties), but he is not a smoker. He does not recall the results of a recent lipid profile. His weight is about 240 lbs., admittedly heavy for his six-foot athletic frame. He exercises only occasionally, as his business schedule precludes a regular exercise regimen. At this point, his wife interjects that his schedule has been especially hectic the past few months with a risk of downsizing in his department and subsequent job-performance stressors.

Upon examining him I notice that his blood pressure is slightly elevated, but otherwise his heart and lung exams are normal. The nurse shows me his electrocardiogram, which I interpret as normal.

I concur that his current lifestyle sounds very stressful. I outline my concerns for potential cardiac pain and initiate a diagnostic work-up that will include a chest radiograph, cardiac enzyme analysis, and a chemical stress test to be completed tonight in the ER. He questions the need for the stress test, but his wife nods approvingly regarding this further diagnostic evaluation. I instruct him to notify the nurse if any pain recurs and am on my way.

Julie S.

This middle-aged woman stares blankly at me as I enter her room. The chart notes her to be having increasing depression in the last few days.

The negative energy in the room is palpable as I interview this woman. Her voice is soft and flat. Her answers are short and terse. She is by herself in the room. Her hair is disheveled, and her clothes are frumpy, dirty, and drab. She smells of stale cigarette smoke. I cannot determine her age by appearance, but when she states that she is thirty-seven I would have easily guessed her to be in her fifties. She is moderately obese.

Despite being medicated with three different antidepressants and a benzodiazepine for breakthrough symptoms, she is still overcome with symptoms of depression and hopelessness. She has no job. Her two children are grown and seldom see her. She has been divorced for three years. She is not suicidal but states little reason for living.

Her physical exam is unremarkable. I try to hide the fact that I cannot wait to get out of her room, but I cannot afford to start the night with this energy-draining encounter. I promise to talk with our social worker to try to get her some better support in the community.

Alice T.

This frail, emaciated woman stares blankly at the wall as I go to examine her. She appears to be quite debilitated with advanced dementia and malnutrition. She does not acknowledge me as I call her name but rather continues dully gazing at nothing in particular. The smell of old urine permeates the room, and the stains of dried feces are evident upon her legs. All of these sensory assaults originate from a loosely fitting diaper. Her body is contorted into a ball as flexure contractures tell a tale of chronic immobility. The mucous membranes lining her mouth and eyes reveal at least moderate dehydration, and her skeletal appearance suggests significant undernourishment. She has a fever and is breathing fast; otherwise, I cannot detect any other acute problem. She is certainly not going to help me with her history or why she was sent here from the nursing home.

Accompanying her chart is a voluminous nursing home record. Recent laboratory tests, radiographs, and physician notes are loosely categorized by date and are of little benefit in elucidating her current problem. Five pages of medications are available for my perusal. Her medications include several cardiac medications, anxiety and depression meds, blood sugar pills, and a cholesterol-lowering drug. It appears that the nursing home staff has found her to be increasingly confused and lethargic over the past two weeks. She has been eating and drinking less and has vomited several times. It seems that the staff is concerned about a recurrent urinary tract infection. This would be her fifth visit to the ER this year for the assessment and treatment of dehydration and infection.

Of most interest to me is her social history. A retired schoolteacher, widowed these past twenty years, she has now been at a nursing home for ten years. Her three children are out of state. The eldest daughter lives in California and acts as the power of attorney. She has requested full resuscitative measures be undertaken for her mother in the case of any illness. It is not clear if she has been made aware of this current transfer.

It is most likely that another infection has loosed itself upon this unfortunate woman. I initiate treatment with intravenous fluids, antibiotics, and blood and urine testing. The nurse promises to try to contact the daughter.

Mike R.

After a quick introduction to this hardened, forty-year-old truck driver, I am assailed with a request for rapid and aggressive pain management. This type of patient is well known to every emergency physician. Little chart review is necessary, as the stories are all remarkably similar. Heavy labor jobs were worked early in life. Then some relatively minor traumatic event unleashed subsequent years of back pain, which surgeries and pain management have done little to alleviate. Now it is a life of constant pain, narcotic dependency, and frequent pain-management encounters. The story this time is back pain exacerbation after helping a friend move into a new apartment. I predict the likelihood of this account being truthful to be exceptionally low. After years of caring for the chronic pain patient, I have abandoned any hope of verifying the reported mechanism of injury. The chronic pain patient's body and mind have been conditioned to function on narcotics, abetted by numerous ER physicians and pain-management specialists.

I find him writhing on the examination cart, clutching his back and grimacing in pain. His vital signs are normal, and his skin is dry. His abdomen is obese. On his lower back are well-healed surgical incisions. There is diffuse tenderness upon palpating his lower back. Despite pain radiating down the back of his legs he has a normal neurological examination.

His medication profile reveals numerous narcotic, antidepressant, and muscle-relaxant medications. He is adamant that none of these are helping his current painful crisis. He states the only thing that helps his pain is Dilaudid injections. I ask him about other therapies he has investigated, but he tells me that nothing else helps when it gets this bad. An analgesic shot is ordered.

Brenda F.

The laughter and squealing emanate down the hallway from this next patient's room. Clearly no serious illness resides here. Excited giggling greets my entrance. There is a young mother with her two children, ages seven and five. There first voice I hear is the five-year-old asking me what is dangling from my neck. This woman and her children have had cold symptoms for several days, and usually an antibiotic helps to clear it right up. There is no reported vomiting, trouble breathing, or headaches from any of them. Mom has been using over-the-counter cough and cold meds with no appreciable benefit.

An examination of ears, throats, and lungs reveal no abnormalities other than slight nasal congestion with discharge. Neither child is able be still during the examination; they are in constant motion. Both mother and children smell of cigarette smoke.

Melissa H.

There is a palpable tension in this next room. A fifty-five-year-old, stylish, well-manicured woman is lying on her right side, grimacing. Her ex-husband stands by her side caressing her shoulder. He does most of the talking, telling me that his ex-wife is suffering from an exacerbation of her fibromyalgia and needs some pain relief. She currently is in a pain-management program, but neither the medications nor the prescribed therapies are working. She is currently not working outside the home, which she now occupies by herself. Her ex-husband is the CEO of a local technology company and travels extensively. Her children are grown, the youngest just having left for college this past month. She has suffered from no recent illnesses other than her fibromyalgia.

Her examination reveals no acute problem other than tenderness in numerous areas on her back, arms, and legs. Her ex-husband continues to stand next to her throughout the exam and is reluctant to let her answer any questions. The patient is quiet and seems depressed. I recommend some IV fluids, laboratory analysis, and analgesics.

Frank L.

The nurse has summoned me emergently to this patient who is brought in by ambulance after an apparent overdose. His mental status has deteriorated en route from his home, and he is now stuporous and obtunded with depressed respirations. The ER team initiates appropriate resuscitative measures, including the administration of Naloxone, an opioid antagonist. The drug caused an immediate improvement in his mentation and awareness, and now he is alert and talking to me. He smells of alcohol. He tells me he took a handful of his mother's Vicodin and drank a six-pack of beer. He was not intending to harm himself; he just wanted to "get high" to escape for a while.

This twenty-year-old tells me that he is currently unemployed and lives at home with his parents. He finished high school but dropped out of the local college after one semester. He spends his days hanging out with friends and is up most nights playing video games. He has been depressed recently but is not suicidal.

I continue his treatment by administering activated charcoal to absorb the Vicodin, and he will be observed in the department for several hours.

Lisa G.

I greet the next patient as she lies in a darkened room clutching a wastebasket from home. The nurses have noted that this is her fourth visit this month for treatment of migraine headaches. I know Lisa well from past visits. She is a divorced mother of four, works long hours as an LPN in a nursing home, has struggled with alcoholism and depression, and is usually brought to the ER by one of her teenage children so that she will have a ride home after her pain shot. It is the same story today. Long days and increased stress have caused another flare-up of her headaches. Despite taking her prescribed medications for migraines and depression, she feels that a pain shot is required for resolution of her symptoms.

As I examine her she describes pain around her scalp on both sides. Her neurologic examination is normal. She is afebrile. I find nothing to suggest that she has meningitis.

In the past we have done numerous CT scans of her brain to assess for hemorrhage, but all of her scans have been normal. Usually she just receives a pain shot and is sent home. I write for her usual cocktail of narcotic and antiemetic therapy and ask the nurse to release her in an hour.

Henry S.

This seventy-year-old looks up from his magazine as I enter the room. He looks pleasant. I think I have seen him before, and he does indeed recognize me. He tells me that his belly pain is acting up again. He tells me that he had another CT scan of his abdomen last week and nothing was found. He has had these pains for years. He has had numerous surgeries done in the attempt to relieve his pain, but despite losing his gallbladder, appendix, and several parts of his colon, nothing has helped him. He is experiencing the same pains as before.

He was a steelworker for years, put his kids through college, and now lives in a retirement home. His wife died about ten years ago, and he lives by himself.

His examination finds him to be resting comfortably. His abdomen has some diffuse tenderness around the umbilicus. There are no abnormal masses. His vital signs are normal.

I promise some narcotic pain relief and order appropriate testing of blood and radiographs to assess for acute abdominal processes. I review his records in our electronic medical records and find an extensive recent medical evaluation. All imaging and laboratory analyses have failed to reveal any abnormalities.

This finishes my first round of patients for the night. These patient scenarios are fabrications. Yet I see them every night. Every emergency physician does. These scenarios, or close variations, are played out in every ER, every day, in our nation's hospitals. Their situations are ubiquitous in our culture. They represent a medical culture in disarray and a society in desperate need of true healing. Let us leave them for a while, step back, and evaluate the causative factors of our health-care crisis.

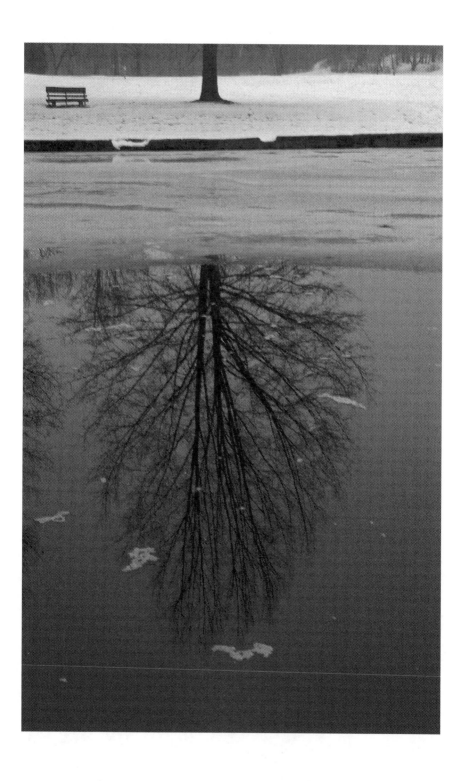

Part I: Disease: Modern Presumptions and Misdirections

The greatest obstacle to progress is not ignorance but the illusion of knowledge.

Daniel Boorstin

Beyond a given point man is not helped by more "knowing" but only by living and doing in a partly self-forgetful way.

Ernest Becker

We currently exist in a culture that is floundering amidst the modern idols of the body and its pleasures and the mind and its distractions. Despite the amazing advances in scientific thought in the past centuries, we are possibly the most perplexed era of people in the history of human discourse. What is one supposed to be doing in this life? Unhappiness pervades the modern world, a deep underlying discontent with the world and the self. How can this be? Leisure time is in abundance, the opportunities for pleasure and comfort abound, and the mysteries of our external world have been tamed.

However, despite a plethora of modern distractions, our world is experiencing an epidemic of ennui. If you are reluctant to admit that our modern disease is despair, then I encourage you to watch any news program, drive through any urban neighborhood, look at the prevalence of modern addictions, engage the diversions of the modern media, or perhaps most revealingly, spend a shift with any ER doctor. Ours is an empty culture, devoid of meaningful dialogue and unwilling to face the realities of the human condition. Most of us are content to be, in the words of T. S. Eliot, "distracted from distraction by distraction."

Let us examine the modern myths that have allowed this modern wasteland to flourish. I will consider four topics that have gradually become ensconced into the modern dialectic:

(1) The predominant worldview is now a materialistic one based on the scientific discoveries of the nineteenth century.

(2) The gradual destruction of societal institutions of authority has elevated the reality interpretations of the individual to become definitive.

(3) Scientism has achieved supremacy in the realm of truth declarations so that there is a complete reliance upon science to give ultimate verification and revelation of truth.

(4) Individuals seek, above all, pleasure and distraction; suffering is seen as anomalous and unnatural.

It is my contention that these beliefs are at best incomplete and at worst incorrect. Modern man needs to rediscover and apply the wisdom of the ages as revealed by some of its wisest teachers.

(1) The Triumph of Materialism

$$E = mc^2$$

Albert Einstein

For those who live according to the flesh set their minds
on the things of the flesh, but those who live according
to the Spirit set their minds on the things of the Spirit.
To set the mind on the flesh is death, but to set the mind
on the Spirit is life and peace.

Paul of Tarsus

Throughout the history of mankind there was thought to be a mysterious
unity of body, spirit, and mind that was coordinated in a mysterious
labyrinth by supernatural means that was referred to as God, YHWH,
Brahmin, and Allah, to name a few titles of the great IS. Then came
the age of enlightenment and rationalism. "I think therefore I am" was
Descartes's rallying cry to a new birth of intellectual freedom for the
human condition. The mind was given reign over the interpretation
of reality. Through the means of rational inquiry the mysteries of the
universe could be explained and conquered. Mind and body are not
mysteriously connected but separate. The course of the last few hundred
years has proven this to be a prescient insight. Think of the progress! In
every area of science great understanding has been achieved regarding
physical reality, leading to inventions that have revolutionized human
life. To this era of progress we owe much gratitude and appreciation.
Material comforts and relative ease of living have never been at a higher
level in those parts of the world that have embraced materialism and
capitalism.

The philosophy of materialism maintains that the natural world is
composed of measurable, quantifiable substances that can be finitely
deconstructed into their ultimately irreducible components. The body
is composed of organ systems that can be reduced to tissues that can be
reduced to cells that can be reduced to organelles that can be reduced
to biochemical substrates and ultimately atoms. The same analysis
can be given to anything in existence. The assumption of science is
that complex structures can be reduced into simple substrates. These
substrates can be measured to give us information about the self and
the world.

Biotechnologies have been developed so that the human body can be imaged very precisely and give very accurate information regarding the status of a body system or organ. Tissues and cellular components can be isolated, extracted, and analyzed to reveal subsequent health or disease that is present. Hematology can isolate and measure blood components that reflect certain disease states. The sequencing of the human genome is revealing the substrates from which cells and organs derive. Subsequently, much disease and suffering has been treated and alleviated. Genetic manipulation harbors a limitless potential of health benefits.

This data can be relied upon to make treatment decisions because this information is thought to accurately reflect the condition of the thing being measured. This is the basis of our modern world of scientific inquiry. We are what our measurements tell us we are. However, these disease processes are the results of causes that remain elusive. Let us not forget that science cannot nor has it claimed to give *ultimate* answers. There are many theories as to the causative factors of certain diseases. Some theories are highly probable. If you smoke cigarettes, then you have a much higher risk of getting cancer than nonsmokers. But many smokers do not get cancer. Why the difference? Science does not know. We do not know why some people get certain diseases and others do not; there are only theories. Certainly there must be other factors involved that are either unrecognizable or immeasurable. Why do the diagnostic tools of the modern physician often fail to give satisfactory clinical answers to many patients' symptoms?

We also stand in the wake of Darwinism, the topic of much modern debate and confusion. Simply stated, Darwin claimed that the macroscopic world changed over the millennia from simpler to more complex in organization as a functional adaptation to the respective organisms' environmental stressors. Modern science has verified Darwin's presumptions (Darwin himself had no knowledge of cellular functions). Genes can mutate or be inserted into existing gene structures, thus creating a new variant of an existing species. This mutation would benefit the organism in a way to increase its chances of survival. This would occur gradually over the course of many years and generations.

(Interestingly, no transitional species have been definitively isolated. Therefore, *interspecies* mutation is still theoretical, while *intraspecies* mutation is definitive.) The simply stated fact is that species change over time to adapt to environmental stressors. This is incontrovertible.

This is all well and good and has been verified by science. In reality, however, this type of analysis tells us little about who we are, from where we came, or what we are supposed to be doing. It cannot explain the intellect, creativity, or the consciousness present in Homo sapiens. It cannot give adequate explanations of first causes. It cannot explain the irreducible complexity of living organisms. It is misleading to claim that Darwinism as a philosophy gives ultimate answers. To claim the philosophy of Darwin as a refutation of a Divine will is irresponsible. To claim a Darwinian worldview is intellectually impoverished. Scientific inquiry is no further along in understanding the human condition than it was before Darwin.

Despite the success of rationalism over the past several hundred years, modern man finds himself adrift in a desperate spiritual wasteland. The quest for meaning for the individual has never been more acute. There seems to be no higher purpose when an ideology of materialism is adopted. According to the evolutionary biologist, our purpose in life is to survive and reproduce. The age of reason and evolution has seen more atrocities perpetrated by man upon other men than any other time in history. The twentieth century is arguably the zenith of man's ability to destroy himself, his cultures, and his world.

If man is allowed to make his own truths based upon rationalism, this seems to be the outcome: a desperate quest for control of the world through conflict, control, and destruction. The ultimate human quest is survival of the particular tribe with which one asserts membership. One needs only to look at the atomic age to argue against materialism, both for the power to destroy and the insight to reveal.

We can dispatch materialism as a worldview quite readily with the coming of modern physics. Because of its abstract complexity it has been avoided by the masses of modern men. Most simply do not believe that an understanding of modern physics is relevant to their daily lives. Perhaps in the egocentrism of our modern, superficial, distracted culture there is no room for this discussion. It is thought to be esoteric and restricted to academia. Actually, it is the basic scientific insight that describes our reality and ultimately explains consciousness, awareness, and the phenomenal world. To better understand man's present quagmire and to facilitate release from false worldview assumptions, this discussion needs to occur in the public arena.

This author does not pretend to be able to discuss modern physics other than in very simple summary statements. To explore the nuclear world is to be quickly enmeshed in abstraction and confusion. Einstein declared the world to be quite different from what Newton described. Newtonian physics remains the foundation of science education and adequately describes physical interactions on the scales in which the majority of our lives are spent. This is the scientific understanding that most people have been given in their public educations. Masses interact in predictable fashions, energy and force are conserved and measurable, and the macroscopic world is ordered. Equations can be utilized to predict and describe interactions between objects in the microscopic world. In short, Newton describes a "clockwork world."

Einstein agreed with Newton when these actions take place on these large scales of measurement. However, scientists in the nineteenth century found phenomena on a much smaller scale that could not be explained by using Newtonian explanations. These perplexities occurred in the subatomic world, the world of electrons, protons, quarks, and neutrinos. The atom, actually, is not the least reducible substance our physical world.

In particular, electrons seemed to behave unpredictably at times. At times the electron could be measured as matter and at other times as energy. These behaviors could not be reconciled with Newtonian physics. Einstein's genius was to propose new theories for the behavior of subatomic particles. Mass and energy are actually involved in an intricate dance in which much is uncertain.

Likewise, the presumed constants of space and time are related to the speed of the relative objects (assuming that speed remains constant). Gravity, always poorly understood, was found to represent the changing of space-time by masses upon other masses. The great insights of Einstein forever changed the Newtonian worldview. Newton's science gives a misleading interpretation of our reality. Quite simply, there is more than meets the eye when one is trying to explain phenomena.

Scientists such as Planck, Einstein, Bohr, Schrodinger, and Heisenberg found the atom to be composed of a mysterious unity of particles and waveforms, an intricate, unknowable dance of energy and mass. They travel throughout the atom in tiny packets called quanta. Heisenberg stated that we have to ultimately accept uncertainty when asking questions about the atom. His experiments revealed that one cannot simultaneously know both the momentum and the position of a subatomic particle. Even more astounding is the fact that whatever an observer looks for—particle or wave—is what will be found. The observer directly influences the result of an experiment. The implications of these revelations are profound.

It can be concluded that the philosophy of materialism as a worldview must be discarded. The material worldview does not reveal an ultimate reality. My patients in the ER who are not in a state of bodily crisis have real pain, despair, and anguish, even though all of the information modern science can give me reveals no abnormality. Something else is going on that we cannot measure.

(2) The Triumph of Individualism

Whoever shall save his life will lose his life.

Jesus of Nazareth

If a man lives, then he must have faith in something.

Tolstoy

Wretched man that I am!

Paul of Tarsus

Two events occurred in the age of enlightenment that severely disrupted the balance of nature and man's perception of his place in the universe. One of these has been discussed—rationalism: the belief that ultimate truths can be reasoned by the intellect. The other occurred through the actions of a German monk, Martin Luther. His rationale was quite reasonable. He saw a corrupt church and wanted to right it. For fifteen hundred years the Catholic Church had dictated and directed daily lives with a combination of "mystery, authority, and magic" as Dostoevsky rightly posits. Holy scriptures were only studied and interpreted by church designees. Truth was revealed through faith, holy scripture, spirit-inspired church leaders, and tradition. The purpose of the individual life was to serve a higher law; thus one's earthly works were of paramount importance in achieving salvation. Subsequent actions and beliefs were subject to review and approval by church canon and priestly authority.

Luther saw this authority suffer from abuses as priests required the payment of indulgences for prayer as the ugliness of the Inquisition swept through Europe. Individual salvation was dependent upon a lifetime of church-sanctioned faith and works. Luther declared that rightness with God occurred with a statement of faith alone. For Luther it was scripture, the grace of God, and faith that gave truth to the individual, not a worldly authority. Individual interpretation of scripture was encouraged.

When the Bible became available to the masses with the advent of the printing press, church authority disintegrated. Modern history is testament to the ensuing chaos. The Western world has been in moral decline ever since the individual was entrusted with scriptural interpretation. As ultimate authority could be discovered and declared by the individual, institutional intervention was no longer necessary.

That has left the individual in a very precarious position. Where does one turn for truth? To science? To scripture? To self? Quantum physics tells us that the world is ultimately unknowable and is subjected to significant bias from individual interpretations of reality. Christian scripture has been removed from the auspices of the church to be placed in the eyes of the beholder and has, through recent scholarship, been found wanting regarding literal reading and interpretation. The self has been found to be a muddied water of self-interest (sin), leaving more questions than answers concerning the purpose of life. How does the modern person define himself?

Thus defines the modern problem: who am I? There exist as many theories regarding human behavior as one would care to study. Why do we act the way we do? Behaviorists, geneticists, Darwinists, sensualists, hedonists, humanists, deists, etc., believe that they know why humans behave as they do. Take your pick. The individual self has been declared the highest authority for making worldview decisions and declarations.

In his revealing book, *The Denial of Death*, Ernest Becker explores the ultimate motivations for human action. To justify oneself, the individual embarks upon a quest for heroism. This is a quest to declare "I am important." To do this the ego coats reality with illusions: my opinions matter; I am unique. Ideally, these illusions are developed within the structure that society has presented for the individual; some role to fulfill that gives one's life purpose and meaning. At some point the problem of life rears its ugly head. Despite a meaningful quest for purpose, the honest man realizes his fate. After years of work, suffering, sacrifice, pleasures, and a sense of uniqueness, his body fails and he dies. To what end? Modern man has no avenues available in which he can transcend the ultimate realities. This has allowed our modern culture of distracted peoples to flourish. What is essential, after all?

The belief that an individual can determine what is best without input from a higher authority has proven to be a fallible assumption. From my perspective as an emergency physician, people are more dysfunctional, unhappy, isolated, and lonely now than ever. Without reliable resources for guidance and authority, the modern world has made idols out of the pursuits of power, pleasure, and possessions. We are awash in information while thirsting for wisdom. There is everywhere a desperate grasping for control as the individual clutches for security and purpose. Every day in my emergency department I see patients/customers who demand treatments of which they know little but have been empowered to expect, even to demand. They believe that they are the ultimate authority regarding their bodies. They are playing with fire.

The triumph of individualism has led directly to a complete erosion of personal responsibility. The individual ego has made an idol of itself; it can do no wrong. When the highest pursuit is to sate desires, then there is no accountability. If there is no accountability for one's actions, then when adversity arises culpability is sought elsewhere. Other individuals or society as a whole is blamed for adverse outcomes. We see this across every level of society. We are a culture of "victims"; a desperate grasping for security in a world that is ultimately mysterious. One needs only to look at our legal system to witness the realities of a "self"-centered culture, our legal system that feeds upon the relativism of truth statements and exists to enrich the attorneys and their clients.

The individual has been empowered to make rational decisions regarding his happiness, welfare, and fate. The problem is that there is no solid foundation upon which to base those decisions. The modern individual has built a house upon sand. We rely on our intellects to make foundational truth declarations and subsequently often develop faulty belief systems.

Thus our current cultural chaos is founded upon a thin veneer of relativism. Each person has been empowered to determine truth. This leads to the modern disease—anxiety. When there is no certain truth other than the very malleable whim of the ego, then worry, fear, and anxiety become the dominant reactions to life stressors and uncertainties.

(3) The Assumption of Certainty

> There is more in heaven and earth than is dreamt of in your philosophy.
>
> Hamlet

For now we see in a mirror dimly, but then face to face.
Now I know in part; then I shall understand fully.

Paul of Tarsus

With the elevation of science and individualism to modern icons it follows that truth can be known. If we can study and measure something, the intellect can make declarative statements of certainty. However, if everyone can be the sole judge of his or her own truth, then we have difficulties if there exist disparities in truth declarations. We do indeed find ourselves in the midst of such difficulties. Individuals tend to make decisions that promote their well-being. The acquisition of safety, comfort, and pleasure becomes paramount. Things or persons that infringe upon these qualities become the opposition and must be eradicated or punished. If my truth is not affirmed, then it is you, not I, who is mistaken. This is relativism, and it describes the state of our modern culture.

Personal responsibility has eroded because the only judge of behavior is the individual. We no longer believe that a life can be led sacrificially. Our legal system unfortunately supports the claim that the perception of the individual must be upheld at all costs. If damage is incurred, it is someone's fault and there must be retribution. We as a culture cannot ignore the fact that potential legal ramifications have forever changed the physician–patient relationship, indeed the workings of all relationships in this "me-first" culture. This is a significant cause of our current health-care crisis and a huge factor in our struggling economy.

Physicians have always known that the body is a mysterious labyrinth, and certainty in diagnosis and treatment is often spurious. Perhaps this truth has become lost in the modern wave of scientism. Certainty cannot be held as a reasonable goal in the practice of medicine. The vast majority of diagnostic tests ordered by physicians are normal or don't alter treatment. Again, most of the tests that are ordered in modern medicine are *medically unnecessary*. This should give us all pause as we face a looming economic crisis and a failing health-care system. Why are these tests ordered?

Our medical delivery systems are being crushed by the quest for certainty. Most patient evaluations involve a search for a disease that is unlikely to be present. This leads to much unnecessary testing and resultant expenditures. The harsh reality of emergency medicine is the fact that most people do not need treatment of any kind; their diseases are self-limited or are of a chronic nature for which medicine has not found an answer. Or there exists some psychic imbalance for which modern medicine can offer no definitive recourse. The best treatment in a surprising number of disease states is actually no treatment. The truths of patients' disease states remain unspoken. The body ages, wears out, and decays, and this vast array of diagnostics and therapies are either of little help or simply allow you, the patient, to avoid confronting the harsh realities of existence, preventing wisdom, resolution, and acceptance.

However, because of current patient expectations (individualism) much testing and treatment is undertaken. If the customer is always right, then the customer decides his own truth (n.b., patients who are suffering a crisis in bodily function do not judge the quality of their respective treatments, for obvious reasons). As a result of such risk-avoidant practices much harm can and does occur. Radiation-induced cancers are developing from the indiscriminate use of diagnostics. Significant morbidity and mortality is induced from the overuse of certain medications (i.e., Warfarin). Many patients suffer from the uncritical use of potentially potent and harmful medications.

The response from many of my colleagues to these criticisms is to laud the successes in longevity we are seeing. People are living longer, healthier lives than ever. Our society needs to have a serious discussion regarding the wisdom of this philosophy. Are the elderly enjoying a fuller quality of life? Are they passing on wisdom to those who follow? To what purposes should one pursue longevity? Pleasure? Increased wealth? More comfort and leisure time?

Do we as a society value the wisdom of the elderly? Have the seasons of life, indeed the circle of life, been recognized by our society? Has the simple fact of acquiring a longer life span become a goal of existence in its own right? At what point does an individual accept fate and acquiesce to the ravages of time? Again, spend a day in a busy ER to witness the effects of achieving longevity without dignity.

Through the ages, physicians have been very comfortable with uncertainty. We have always known that the mysteries of this world cannot be predicted or diagnosed with certainty in the majority of disease processes. Physical manifestations of disease have various causes originating in the immaterial realm. All we can ever do is give probabilities as to the presence of disease.

In the past, physicians have been able to help patients achieve dignity in disease and in death by helping them seek greater realities and wisdom as their diseases progressed. Now there is an endless seeking for quantity of life as opposed to quality, wisdom, or transcendence of our earthly existence. There is an absolute expectation that life's sufferings can be met and overcome through the utilization of scientific investigation and treatment.

True, modern technologies have increased diagnostic accuracy. But every physician knows that uncertainty still lurks. The modern clinician is still left with theory and presumption when the results of diagnostic testing yield no definitive answer. And this happens with increasing frequency in modern medical practice.

The stakes are now much higher in the practice of medicine. Missed diagnoses are now punishable by lawsuits and dismissals from hospital staffs or physician groups. Physician discontentment is at an all-time high. The majority of diagnostic tests that are ordered either have normal outcomes or do not significantly impact therapy. This fact is leading our medical system into financial ruin. Certainty is not attainable for any length of time. Our culture has an unreasonable expectation of certainty.

Modern physics asserts that certainty is not possible. Phenomena may be altered by the observer and by the nature of the world. As the analysis of the self has shown, reliable knowledge of the self is limited and usually directed at self-contentment. Upon what exactly does one base decision-making regarding care? Should one consider long-term or short-term results? Should one consider the group as a whole, or simply the individual, when making health-care decisions? The best we can hope for is certitude. One is forced at some point to ask what is really known with certainty in the human mind. All stimuli are filtered through the individual mind fully equipped with its experience, senses, perceptions, and subsequent judgments. We are simply unable to see clearly when the individual's focus is on his own needs and desires.

In the wake of modern scholarship, much aspersion has been cast upon the assumptions of truth proclaimed in the world's sacred writings. Our situation is not hopeless, but it is chaotic. Can we know anything with certainty? Ourselves? Our world? I have found that critics of sacred writings have seldom spent much time in contemplative reflection upon their words. The converse is also true. Many people who are devoutly religious seldom cast a critical eye upon the sacred writings of their faith. Pontius Pilate famously asked Jesus, "What is Truth?" That question is as relevant today as it was two thousand years ago. As a result of years of truth-seeking, I claim to only assert probabilities and not certainties. The ultimate reality simply is. It cannot be defined. It is probable that we understand very little about the ultimate reality of our lives or experiences.

(4) The Denial of Suffering

> When you are living in darkness, why don't you look for the light?
>
> The Dhammapada

> Modern man is drinking and drugging himself out of awareness, or he spends his time shopping, which is the same thing.
>
> Ernest Becker

The most memorable opening line of any book I have read is from Scott Peck's *The Road Less Traveled*: "Life is difficult." A succinct, honest, and declarative summary statement. It is a truth lost upon much of the Western world. The successes of science notwithstanding, life remains rife with challenges, hurdles, and psychic and physical pain. I contend that modern science will do little to alleviate the psychic sufferings of man. The use of psychotropic medication is now commonplace in our morass of mass societal dysfunction. Is the commonplace use of these medications augmenting or suppressing the human experience? Pharmacotherapy may quiet the beast for a short while, but the beast will not be tamed so easily. Physical suffering will always occur. Psychic pain is ubiquitous. The role of the modern-day physician is to treat pain aggressively and indiscriminately. The great question remains: to what purpose is suffering? Pain is a valuable teacher. It warns of bodily disease. It instructs the sufferer to rest while healing occurs. As a daily companion it can lead to greater truths. Suffering must lead us to a greater truth as a community as well.

The acceptance of pain stands in direct conflict to the modern understanding of personal fulfillment. We define our positions in the world and justify our existences by what we do, what we earn, what material goods we acquire, what we enjoy. Suffering occurs when we are denied the acquisition of these modern ego-definitions and is subsequently viewed as an anomaly. Suffering is construed as a personal failure, success denied.

There is a great paradox in life. Despite a world full of beauty, joy, and pleasure, we are plagued by pain, tragedy, and death. There exists evil amidst the good. The existence of suffering has been the subject of theological debate for centuries. There has not been a consensus as to why suffering exists, but we do not want for suppositions.

The Book of Job in the Old Testament provides the best of any answers. Suffering simply exists, and it is not for us, in this human arena of existence, to know the why or wherefore. Perhaps we are being disciplined for wrong behavior. Maybe our perseverance is being tested. We may suffer because of choices we have made. It all may represent some cosmic battleground in which we are simply pawns. Job learns that all ultimately is mystery, for we mortals cannot possibly understand the mind of the Divine.

Ironically, the great sages all look to suffering as the key to wholeness. It is through the confrontation of suffering that we ultimately find truth and redemption. (This should not be construed to minimize suffering in any way. I have seen great suffering in the ER. Individual suffering is real. It may, however, be more accurate to state that the perception of pain is real.)

We moderns do not put much thought into the problem of evil. Why do bad things happen? We have too many distractions to consider this seriously. From my experiences in the ER, I can tell you that few people are prepared to deal with these issues. If one has not considered these issues during times of comfort, then in times of crisis there will be despair and confusion. Why do bad things happen to good people? Indeed, why do bad things happen at all?

We as a culture are failing in our attempts to quell suffering with various forms of escapism, diversion, and distraction. The increased use of psychotropic pharmaceutical agents is failing in the attempt to alleviate psychic sufferings or sustain people through the difficulties that life brings. The tried-and-true methods of escape through chemical addictions, however, continue to thrive. The modern descent into mediocrity is fueled by modern media's ability to consume the human psyche with inanities. Boredom is not allowable in our current market, designed to distract the modern ego into oblivion.

Suffering must be acknowledged and confronted, individually and collectively. It is insanity to pretend that suffering has been conquered, controlled, or tempered. Just because physical suffering can be anaesthetized does not mean that there is any less psychic or communal suffering. And a lack of awareness of the sufferings of others does not excuse one from action.

In the East there is a belief in karma. Karma maintains that one's actions or inactions cause effects in this or in following lifetimes, based upon the relative goodness of the actions. If there is positive, it will result in more positives; if negative, then there will occur more negatives.

Karmic laws can teach us about the manner in which we confront suffering. One can endure and overcome suffering and thus remove oneself from the karma that ensues. One can continue to accrue more suffering if one maintains a path that attracts these negative emotions, actions, or beliefs.

There is also a balance that exists in our experiences. Good and evil are always present, and one or the other will predominate personally or collectively at certain times in life. There will be light and dark, strong and weak, masculine and feminine, joy and despair. Ours is a world of contrasting opposites. This is known as the yin and yang principle in China. Despite our best intentions, there will always be a balance of these forces in the self and in others. It is therefore imperative that we escape from our Western preoccupations with pleasure, ease, and comfort and face the reality that has always challenged human existence.

Suffering *is*.

The Culture of Desire

Selfish desire is found in the senses, mind, and intellect, misleading them and burying the understanding in delusion.

The Bhagavad Gita

There is nothing good or bad, but thinking makes it so.

Hamlet

Take heed, and beware of all covetousness; for a man's life does not consist in the abundance of his possessions.

Jesus of Nazareth

The ideologies of materialism and individualism have induced our current milieu of a culture enmeshed in escapism. We seek escape from our realities in the distractions of modern media, drug addiction, sex, gluttony, greed, the pursuit of worldly success, envy, and despair. The human self is collapsing upon itself in a ceaseless quest to satisfy its desires. Without a higher authority in which to lose oneself in service, modern man pursues endless distractions to fill himself with meaning. These distractions are transient, void of authenticity, and ultimately empty. The self finds itself not filled at all and goes looking for the next diversion. The pleasure that is found ends up leaving the pursuer simply wanting more.

Shakespeare remains eternally relevant because he eloquently summarizes the human condition in his plays and sonnets. His writings remove the layers of illusion that coat man's worldly existence to reveal dark, sobering truths. Consider Sonnet 129 and his description of human desire:

> The expense of spirit in a waste of shame
> Is lust in action; and till action, lust
> Is perjured, murd'rous, bloody, full of blame,
> Savage, extreme, rude, cruel, not to trust;
> Enjoy'd no sooner but despised straight;
> Past reason hunted; and no sooner had,
> Past reason hated, as a swallow'd bait,
> On purpose laid to make the taker mad:
> Mad in pursuit, and in possession so;
> Had, having, and in quest to have, extreme;
> A bliss in proof, and proved, a very woe;
> Before, a joy proposed; behind, a dream.
> All this the world well knows; yet none knows well
> To shun the heaven that leads men to this hell.

I have never read a better synopsis of the plight of mankind. Who has not felt this predicament? I think Shakespeare's sonnet can be read as a condemnation of human desire in general, not simply sexual lust. Any indiscriminant, unexamined pursuit of the senses will end in madness.

Our capitalist system cultivates desire. Indeed, it needs consumers with insatiable desires to feed its massive appetite. Our economy suffers when consumerism diminishes. One needs only a few minutes of any typical television or magazine viewing to be subject to a barrage of advertising with the sole aim of inciting our desires. Desires are enflamed for food, sex, medication, cars, comfort, alcohol, and travel so that the unawake viewer is soon nothing more than a vacuous vessel of indiscriminant desire. In fact it would be easy to live a life enmeshed in the unmitigated pursuit of pleasure. Many people do just that. An analysis of the thought life finds that the majority of one's waking hours are spent thinking about things, persons, or experiences that are desired. This would be the unexamined life.

It is my contention that desires consume and define the modern life. We crave many things: money, success, sex, travel, food, drink, possessions, comfort, leisure, control, power, etc. The inherited concept of sin is one of immoral and injudicious action reflecting the individual will in direct opposition to the Divine. There is a moral law, and it reflects the Divine will that lives within us all.

Each of us inherently knows and recognizes "wrong" behavior. The definition of moral behavior did not start upon Mt. Sinai with Moses. Whenever man became aware of good and evil is when the awareness developed of proper behavior. Whether we take the Genesis account of human intellectual development as literal or allegorical, at some point there arose an awareness of moral behavior. And remember, the precursor of action is thought. If thoughts are consumed by desires, then desires will drive action.

Are desires evil unto themselves? There are religious philosophies that denounce any bodily pleasure or worldly pursuits. I contend that many desires are glimpses into the divine when appropriately pursued and enjoyed. We cannot deny the existence of many worldly pleasures. There are undoubtedly many good things in life. When engaged to excess or engaged inappropriately, however, desires control, disparage, torment, and ultimately destroy the life of man. When one pursues pleasure at the expense of another, or when the pursuit of desires lead us away from "the good," then one is pursuing a false god.

Each of us has experienced, at one time or another, desire denied. The emotional, physical, and spiritual pain that results is acute, as all can attest. It is now for us to examine how the inappropriate pursuit of desires can affect the body and its functions. Certainly they do. Remember how one responds when asked to speak in public. Or when one experiences a relational crisis or suffers the loss of a loved one, or even a job. Physical, sexual, and emotional abuses are epidemic in our society. These involve damaging forces that need to be managed by the victim as well as the abuser. It is clear that there are powerful energies at work. Is it possible that these energies manifest in bodily illness? How are these energies related to disease?

The Paradigm Shift

> In order to arrive at what you do not know, you must go by a way which is the way of ignorance.
>
> T. S. Eliot

> Give me that man that is not passion's slave and I will wear him in my heart's core, aye, in my heart of heart.
>
> Hamlet

Let us now return to my patients in the ER. They have all been evaluated appropriately with modern laboratory and radiographic studies and received relevant pharmaceutical intervention. They have not been found to be experiencing a crisis in organic functioning; therefore, the tools at my disposal are reduced to theory and presumption. I cannot give them an authentic diagnosis, nor can I offer them healing. What can we do?

We reevaluate our theory of disease. It is the premise of this book that our current understanding of disease is incomplete. We need to pursue a deeper understanding of our being. Remember where we have been in our recent cultural analysis: ideologically floundering amidst materialism, rationalism, and individualism. We live in a culture that fosters the pursuit of pleasure and ego-gratification as the ultimate purpose of human existence. Moderns are completely ill-equipped to emotionally deal with the inevitabilities of physical and psychic suffering. We need to return to the great questions: Who am I? What am I supposed to be doing? What is the good life? Where am I going? What is ultimate reality? Where do my thoughts originate? The Trappist monk and mystic Thomas Merton has summarized our position:

> We are all too ready to believe that the self that we have created out of our more or less inauthentic efforts to be real in the eyes of others is a "real self." We even take it for our identity. Fidelity to such a nonidentity is of course infidelity to our real person, which is hidden in mystery. Who will you find that has enough faith and self-respect to attend to this mystery and to begin by accepting himself as unknown? God help the man who thinks he knows all about himself.

The great thinkers have always known that we are not what we think we are. There is an ultimate reality, however, that can be pursued and realized. Human life has meaning when it is seeking that which is greater than one's self. Our modern ideologies have failed us.

Modern physics has verified what the mystics of every culture have always known. We humans are a complex, mysterious matrix of mind, body, and spirit. To deny the existence of any of these will lead to an incomplete human. We are not just composed of chemicals, tissues, and organs. This is a description of the surface.

We interact with the spiritual realm in mysterious ways. Our habits of thinking affect us in very real ways. We can learn to impact our physical realities by becoming aware of our inner lives. Thoughts are energies. The spiritual realm is composed of different energies than our physical manifestations. Ultimately all is energy—energy that can be controlled and manipulated to attain maximal health through a transformation of our habits in thought and action; energies that exist in the spiritual realm that can be accessed and utilized for health and healing, not only for ourselves but also for those in our spheres of influence.

My patients should not despair. If they are willing to alter their view of themselves and their world, they will have opened a vista of unlimited resources for better health. In the words of the apostle Paul, "Do not be conformed to this world but be transformed by the renewal of your mind, that you may prove what is the will of God, what is good and acceptable and perfect." This is the road to healing.

It is for us now to reexamine what it means to be in the world. If we denounce the modern understanding of man as material and the individual as authoritative, then we need to look deeper for explanations. The shift in thinking that needs to occur is from the idea that the body is all that exists to accept the position that we are mind, body, and spirit joined in a composite trinity. Yes, we are material beings in this sphere of existence, but ultimately we are energy, a spiritual, living, unified essence.

It is now that we begin a new understanding of health and wellness. We rediscover a timeless understanding of ourselves so that a new paradigm for health may be realized. We must learn that the body responds to our patterns of thinking and our spirit communes with the Divine.

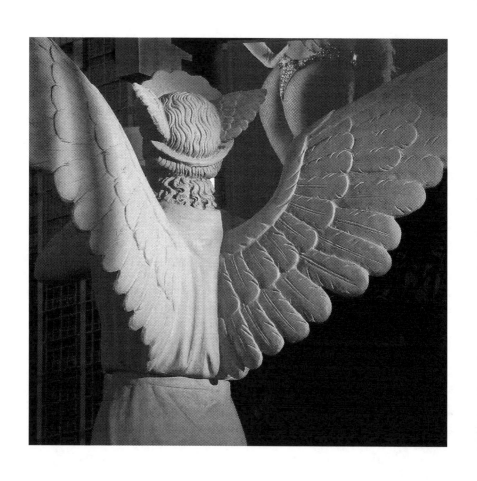

Part II: The Pursuit of Self-Knowledge

There are only hints and guesses, hints followed by guesses; and the rest is prayer, observance, discipline, thought, and action.

T. S. Eliot

What do you seek?

Jesus of Nazareth

Those who are motivated only by the fruits of their action are miserable, for they are constantly anxious about the results of what they do.

Bhagavad Gita

To believe that we are composed of energies, we have to first of all accept the insights of modern physicists and ancient sages and secondly begin to awaken to a different understanding of ourselves. It needs to be understood that our minds, our inner lives, are the vehicle through which this understanding will come. We need to develop an awareness of our separate components—mind, body, and spirit.

I have found few insights from modern psychology or psychiatry. The modern thinking seems to be that we are sensory organisms that have responded to stimuli to create an illusion of separateness. The modern psychiatrist believes that by manipulating our neurochemistry, individual behavior can be positively altered for a happier, more complete life experience; that the human is a conglomeration of chemicals that can be accessed through the use of pharmaceuticals. Can our understanding of the human be reduced to such a shallow doctrine? What exactly is the self?

If we are more than simply material existing solely to seek pleasure and to produce offspring, then we need to explore what else we are or can be. We need to study the teachings of the masters. There is a reason that the writings of the great teachers have been treasured for millennia. They contain great truths. Remember that our current goal is to see the interactions of mind, body, and spirit in maintaining health. First, let us learn about this most confusing of creatures, the individual self. I have found the most insightful teachers to be those who have become the center of spiritual movements; all else is interpretation and commentary.

Jesus of Nazareth

For nearly two thousand years Jesus of Nazareth has proven to be a font of wisdom and transcendence. Yet, as a student of the New Testament Gospels it is not clear to me who Jesus was, or is. To understand the modern world and the evolution of the individual in society, we must examine the message of Jesus as it is given to us in the New Testament Gospel accounts. No one has had a more profound effect on the history of mankind than this first-century Galilean. I find it inexcusable to live in our world and not have read the accounts of his life and teachings. Ultimately one may reject his teachings, but it is irresponsible to condemn the modern church without a serious reading of the Gospels. People were attracted to Jesus in his day because he manifested great power and truth. The same is true today for us modern seekers of truth.

Who is the Jesus of history? Claims are made for a Divine birth, an adoption into the Divine realm, an existence lived as mainly spirit, an incomplete attainment of the Divine nature, and simply a Jewish prophet or teacher. Modern scholars see him as an apocalyptic preacher. Christian doctrine attests that Jesus was born, lived, died, and was resurrected as the unique Son of God and was to be subsequently worshiped as the

Divine reality through which the believer has salvation. He used the monikers Son of Man, Son of God, and Messiah. It is not clear to whom these titles were addressed. None of these terms has an accepted definition in the ancient world in which Jesus lived and taught.

I don't believe that Jesus knew he was anything more than enlightened. Certainly greater minds than mine have struggled with the same question. The ambiguity of Jesus's true identity remains the enigma of the Christian faith. The central mystery of Christian faith is the claim of an atoning death and the subsequent paschal miracle. The Gospel accounts state that Jesus was aware that he would be killed, sacrificed to atone for the sins of many, and would overcome his death, as the Gospels relate.

But which Jesus? The human man who lived, breathed, walked, and preached as the Son of Man, or the Son of God, a person of elevated consciousness, who was equal, or identical to, the Divine?

Who or what exactly is the Son of Man? Who did Jesus interpret himself to be? This seems to me unclear at best. The fulcrum of Mark's Gospel occurs when Jesus asks his disciple Peter, "Who do you say that I am?" The question is as relevant today as it was then.

The Gospel accounts were written decades after he lived and are clearly infused with polemic, encouraging a certain interpretation of this man's life, written for particular communities. To be immersed in these accounts, however, is to be confronted with varying degrees of ultimate truth. Whoever authored these narrative works were certainly witness to some form of elevated teaching, revelation, and transcendence that was full of charisma, power, and truth. All modern Christian scholarship fails to give ultimate answers. The multiplicity of Christian denominations attests to the ambiguity that exists.

What is contested is his message. Is it contained in the modern Protestant view of salvation through faith in Jesus Christ, the historical person who was both fully man and fully Divine? Is Jesus to be worshipped? Does he show us an esoteric, mystical path to enlightenment? What is the modern presupposition of faith?

It seems to me that Jesus teaches salvation through the attainment of the Kingdom of God, an attainment of the consciousness that he was able to embody. This may be what the early Gospel writers meant when referring to faith. The modern church preaches Christ as the center of the message, where it seems to me that Jesus means for the Kingdom to be at the center of the message. The realization of this Kingdom-consciousness appears to go through the same spiritual path that Jesus traveled and is now available to us all through the Holy Spirit. ("The only way to the Father is through the Son.")

The role of Jesus's sacrificial death in the attainment of this consciousness is a deep mystery. It is implied that full acquisition of this transcendent consciousness can occur through the acquisition of the Christ-consciousness. This has somehow been made available to us through the death of the Son of Man—again, mystery shrouded in mystery. A dramatic transcendence from the ego-self to the unity found in Kingdom-consciousness can be realized. ("He who will save his life will lose his life.") The individual perception of personality is completely left behind as one gradually (or suddenly, as in Paul's case) acquires access to knowledge of the Kingdom. For the Christian it is the person of Jesus who represents the Kingdom.

The Gospel of Mark, the first Gospel text to have been written, is a dramatic, fast-paced journey from declaration of the Kingdom to death of the physical body of Jesus of Nazareth on a cross. Jesus's first recorded words are included: "The time is fulfilled; the Kingdom of Heaven is at hand. Repent and believe in the Gospel." This is profound and encapsulates the Kingdom message. We have constant access to the Kingdom. We have to awaken to its presence. Repent—change your thinking. Believe. Believe in what? Jesus as God? No. Believe that the concept of time as we have been taught is now different in this state of Christ-consciousness, and by changing your thinking you can attain Kingdom-consciousness. Repent means to change one's thinking, to rethink. (Rethink what?) The pre-passion Gospel that was preached was Kingdom-directed, not Christ-directed.

Having read and studied the Gospels and the Pauline epistles, I had to erase most of my inherited and learned assumptions about Jesus. Many of the questions asked in the above paragraphs will not have answers in this lifetime. One must become very comfortable with uncertainty and doubt in the pursuit of understanding. I feel strongly that we moderns have inherited a Christian tradition that is incorrectly Christ-focused and that the message that Jesus preached was Kingdom-focused. To change this perception of the Christ is very difficult (another paradigm shift) but is essential to spiritual growth.

Jesus displays his transcendent consciousness through healings, miracles, exorcisms, and esoteric teaching ("Those who have ears ..."). He is simultaneously seen as a healer, revolutionary, radical, social activist, teacher, and sacrificial lamb. He has access to energies to transform physical appearances. He has learned mastery of the self. Indeed, this is his teaching to his disciples. Take up your cross daily— the cross that leads to death of the outer, unenlightened self. Save your life by losing your life, losing the concept that you are simply body, emotions, and thoughts. Find your real life by accessing the Kingdom through the realization of "Christ-consciousness." Access and realize the enlightened consciousness, and one's personal needs and desires will be demoted and ultimately extinguished.

One can access the Kingdom through prayer, humility, and nonattachment to worldly values. This entails great suffering, for the ego does not want to release its claim of superiority. Jesus had to be cleansed of these ego requirements by enduring forty days in the wilderness and afterward being subjected to demonic temptations (see Matt. 4:1–11, Luke 4:1–13). This is the central hurdle in accessing and understanding the Kingdom. The individual must be completely cleansed of all identifications with the ego. Your understanding of yourself must be erased so that you can be filled with the will of God.

As a physician I am intrigued with the healing of the paralyzed man. He was lowered by his friends through the roof to see Jesus (Mark 2:1–12). The man clearly had come to Jesus to be healed. Jesus responded to this request by telling this man that his sins are forgiven! What a surprise this must have been for the sick man to hear! It seems that Jesus believed that the psychic pain this man was harboring from past sin(s) was causing him physical disease and by releasing him from this pain—this energy!—he would be free from disease. The incident of course continued by relating the subsequent conflict with the Pharisees, but it could have easily ended with this forgiveness of sins. Could the psychic pain retained from past unresolved, unrepentant, unforgiven sin—murder, adultery, lying, anger, etc. (inappropriate desires!)—have led directly to physical disease? Jesus apparently thought so.

Even more disturbing to the modern mind is the healing of disease through exorcism (Mark 1:21–27; 5:1–13; 9:14–29). Could this be possible today with our understanding of mental illness? Based upon my experiences in the ER seeing hundreds of patients maintained on antipsychotic and antidepressant medications yet who continue to manifest psychosis, I would maintain that demonic involvement (negative energies, if you prefer) must at least be entertained. We do not have a more plausible explanation.

Could Jesus heal simply by touching , or being touched by another person? Could healing occur even if he was in the vicinity of the diseased person? It seems that he had access to energies or to power that could heal. He had attained a higher consciousness. Be assured that presumptive miracles occur even today. Cancers disappear, chronic pain leaves, infections resolve inexplicably. There is much yet to be learned.

Jesus leads the blind to a gradual awakening through the loss of a worldly identity to a fullness achieved by losing one's understanding of one's self. Jesus gives us access to nourishment that feeds the body and soul. The great paradox—we are found when we lose ourselves. We realize ourselves when we become aware of the Kingdom and seek its fruits.

The first miracle in John's Gospel account tells of the changing of water into a fine wine. This is why we come to Christ, to be purified in our wills and spirits just as the water was purified. We seek the purity of the Christ-consciousness. His teachings, even in a supposedly "post-Christian" world, remain relevant and life changing.

The Buddha

Born into a wealthy family and living a life of comfort and pleasure, Siddhartha looked for a deeper meaning in his life. Despite his comfortable existence he still could not find happiness. He sought the wisdom of the wisest men of the East, he traveled, he read, and still he was no further in finding the secret to life. He finally turned his vision inward. His great insight was to see that the root cause of his sufferings was the existence of desire, desire that was insatiable. To extinguish desire we needed to transform our inner lives. We needed to change our thinking. When desires were overcome one achieved Nirvana—an existence free from suffering.

To maintain a reverence for life, to practice generosity, to exhibit responsible sexual behavior, to speak and listen deeply, and to eat only wholesome substances were habits that would extinguish an individual's desire, and he would suffer no more. Selfishness leads to suffering. All that we are is a result of what we have thought. Meditate. Discipline your mind. Avoid paths that lead to profit and pleasure. Above all, awaken yourself to the lies of this world so that you can be a light to others. When you have neither likes nor dislikes, then you will be free. We are free when we escape from the imprisonment of our thinking. (This all sounds familiar, doesn't it?)

The Buddha leads us to awareness that the sufferings of this world are illusory, created by our ego to sustain the ego's ability to define itself. When we escape these ego delusions we are able to move past the desires of this world to attain the peace and joy that ironically come with this detachment. This state of transcendent peace and joy is called Nirvana. (n.b.: This blissful state that the spiritual masters describe is the same in all religions. Whether one refers to the Kingdom of Heaven or Nirvana, one is talking about the same transcendent state of existence.)

Krishna

For many years I was deeply puzzled by the Protestant dogma of salvation by faith. I seemed to be no different after "accepting Christ" than before making a proclamation of faith. What was I missing? There had to be more to the message of Christ than just uttering a few words. What did "faith" entail?

Ironically, my first understanding of Jesus's teachings came through my readings of the Bhagavad Gita, an ancient Hindu text. In it we are told of an Indian battle long ago in which the young warrior Arjuna is being instructed by the Divine manifested in the person of Krishna. To read the teachings of Krishna is to have the teachings of Jesus come to life. To read about the definition of an illumined man in the second chapter of the Gita is to grasp the deep implications of the Sermon on the Mount in Matthew's Gospel.

Krishna sees the wise as having renounced selfish desires and reveals a deep unity in all of life. Once established in meditation one is freed from lust, fear, and anger. The wise are indifferent to worldly successes or failures. The wise subdue their senses and keep their minds absorbed in the Kingdom of God. A mind united with the Divine will is at rest in peace and joy. To free the senses from attachment is to live in wisdom. What the world calls the day, the wise call the night. To be united with the Lord is the supreme state. Krishna contends that the supreme reality stands revealed in the consciousness of those who have conquered themselves.

Krishna continues in the Gita to expound the virtues of ego-renunciation, selfless service, meditation, and love. To be absorbed in the Gita is to be absorbed in truth. The teachings of the Gita are what have been left out of the modern Christian message. My approach to faith, religion, and exclusionary belief systems has been forever changed by my readings of this wonderful text. There exists a deep and profound unity in this realm of being. Although the prism separates the light into many beautiful colors, there still exists only one light. Krishna, more than any other seer (God? prophet? transcendent? Buddha? yogi?) has brought me to a clearer understanding of the illusions of the self.

The Tao

Reportedly written by Lao-Tzu circa 500 BCE, the Tao presents the reader with a fascinating realization: to know we must not-know. If we can describe or tell of something, then that is not the essence of the thing we are describing. The unnameable is the eternal real. If we free ourselves from desire, we realize the mystery. If we are caught in desire, we see only the manifestations. These short chapters require much careful consideration. These teachings are truly the antithesis to the rationalism and intellectualism that the Western mind deifies.

To be able to name and describe an object is to immediately diminish it and make it unknowable. "Darkness within darkness, the gateway to understanding." The text is at the same time illuminating and inexplicable, very much like life. To enter the pages of the Tao is to greet a barrage of absurdities. To become wise we must unlearn. Light is found in darkness. True action lies in stillness. True leadership involves empowering the people to lead themselves.

The essential message of the Tao is in accord with the other masters. True happiness is found in diminishment. Simplicity, patience, and compassion are essential virtues. We find peace when desire is extinguished. Returning to the source we find serenity. Hope and fear are both phantoms of the mind. Once again we have found a central unity of teaching into the essence of living a good life.

From Medieval to Modern

It would be a Herculean undertaking to try to summarize two millenia of human philosophical endeavors. Certainly one can pursue this if so interested. I have made a cursory attempt to familiarize myself with the great ideas of our past and present. Many great thinkers and writers throughout the years have written and spoken on these very topics we are discussing. Why is it then that the great religious teachers remain so relevant? Have we really learned little more of pertinence regarding the human self in the past two millenia? It is beyond the scope of my current purpose to explore this question. My personal conclusion is to reiterate the eternal relevance of the great spiritual teachers. In seeking truth, the path always has led me back to the great spiritual teachers. Do the well-known and widely studied philosophers have something to add to the debate? Most certainly they do. But it all seems to me as commentary to the teachings of the masters.

Interestingly, during my spiritual quest into the nature of healing, I found several books that had been written by modern sages regarding just these truths. They have been met with explosive popularity by the general public. Having read and enjoyed many of these, I nevertheless have concluded that they add little to the wisdom revealed by these aforementioned ancients.

I also spent quite a bit of time reading the works of recent truth-seekers Jung and Freud. They both explored the psyche for clues of ultimate reality. Despite an unprecedented descent into the subconscious of man, Freud did not get beyond the self and its desires. Jung found in the unconscious mind a mysterious labyrinth of personalities embedded in the myths and wisdoms of the past, much of it revealed in our dream life. The ego-manifestations cover deep layers of mystery, unity, and universality. Truth is unchanging at a very deep and universal level of consciousness. Should these layers be uncovered?

Where does this leave us regarding our road to healing? The great teachers have shown us much. To begin to heal one must begin with knowledge of the self, and this knowledge lies in reexamining the perceptions of who we are. What is described as a particular individual is actually referring to combination of a physical body with senses, emotions, desires, and an intellect. This self is defined by the information it has received from the outer world. It has processed this information based upon perceptions, theories, and conditionings that it has received over a lifetime given to us through our families, cultures, and pasts.

This is a person's life—past experiences and future worries and expectations, which may or may not come to fruition. The moment, the very real, the eternal Now, is lost amidst the concerns of the past and the anxieties over the future. We have learned that this definition of self is false and temporal. To live with this perception of self is to live in despair and unhappiness, because this perception will be made up of desires fulfilled, expected, denied, and regretted. There is an ultimate reality that lies beyond these temporal perceptions and manifestations. Discovering the road to this reality is the road to recovery and true healing.

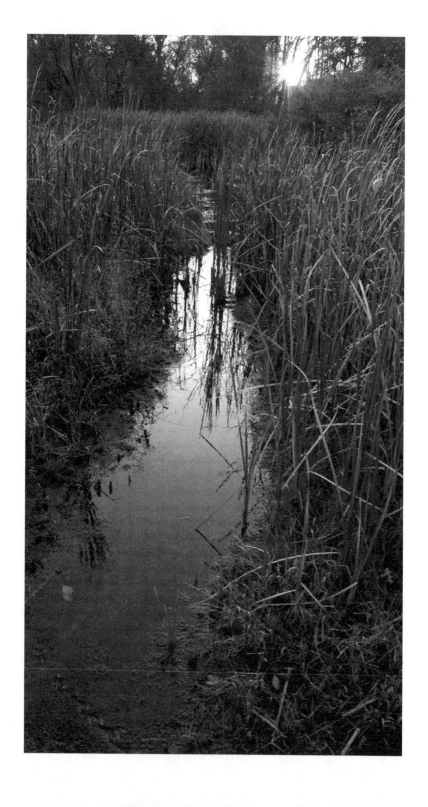

Part III: Spirit and Energy

As salt dissolves in water, so the self dissolves in the Eternal.

Hindu proverb

All of the body is in the mind; not all the mind is in the body.

Swami Rama

We are spiritual beings having a human existence.

Teilhard de Chardin

What is essential is invisible to the eye.

Saint-Exupery

It is now time to awaken to this other dimension of our temporal existence, our spirit and our latent energies. Spirit as understood by moderns is at best nebulous. Are spirit and soul similar or the same? There certainly seems to be some intangible substrate upon which our physical bodies are shaped (the soul?), yet there also exists energies that are both localized individually and apparently universally (the spirit?). I have not found a consensus among philosophers or theologians in describing these most intangible aspects of our beings.

What can be declared is that there is an aspect of being that is eternal, alive, universal, immaterial, and mysterious. The Orient has been a font of wisdom regarding this journey of spiritual awakening. We have seen how the West has influenced the modern advances in technology and science with a rational pursuit and acquisition of knowledge regarding our physical world. We need to rediscover the East and its wisdom regarding our latent energies and intuitions.

As a Western-trained and educated physician I approached the claims of mystics, energy researchers, and healers with skepticism until I tested their claims and was able to personally experience the reality of these energies. What is claimed is that there is a dynamic, vibrating energy field within our physical bodies. There is an extension of this field outside our bodies in an aura of energy. This field of energy can be seen by clairvoyants and be felt by nearly everyone. This energy is described as Qi or prana in the East, and as spirit or life force in the West. There exists an unlimited supply of this energy in the universe. It can be accessed and controlled by the intentional aspirant. How does one develop awareness of and an accession to these energies?

The individual's energy field can be felt and manipulated by using the breath in a controlled fashion. Deep, regulated inspiration with a brief holding of the breath for several seconds, followed by a slow, controlled exhalation, should induce a sense of energy being pulled up into your upper body. It is difficult to describe the actual sensation. I feel a sense of peace, a pulsating rhythm that can be felt in the thoracic area. As one progresses in the realization of these energies, a sense of energies can be felt throughout the body and can actually be intentionally directed to one part of the body or another. As a novice it will take patience, awareness, and practice to feel these energies. During these exercises the mind should be focused on the breath, pulling air down into the diaphragm and feeling the energies concentrate in different parts of the body.

Another energy-awakening exercise is to feel the energy ball formed by your hands. Place your hands in front of you as if you were going to hold a basketball at mid-chest level. Slowly draw the hands away from one another and then back together. At some point you should feel a subtle sense of pulling and pushing as if there were a magnetic field in the vicinity. The easiest and most definitive demonstration of energy is to point your index finger at the palm of your opposite hand. Draw a letter on your palm using your index finger at a distance of several inches. There should be a definitive sensation of energy.

Energy moves in predictable patterns in the balanced, healthy human body. Chakras are energy points in the body that can be easily felt and act as central points where healing can occur. (The word chakra is derived from a Sanskrit word meaning "wheel.") The seers of ancient India first recognized these energy vortices and described them in the Vedic scriptures. Indeed, the energy felt at each chakra can be seen and sensed to be moving in a circular fashion, usually clockwise (think of a clock sitting on your chest for the appropriate directional sense). It has been claimed that by opening the chakras one can access different psychic states, attain supernatural powers, and experience various levels of transcendence. For our current purposes, we will see how the chakras can be accessed to achieve and maintain health and wellness.

There are seven main chakras. There are many other minor chakras. The major chakras are crown, brow (third eye), throat, heart, solar plexus, sacral, and base. It is of no minor coincidence that each chakra corresponds to an endocrine gland, a plexus of nerves, and a collection of lymph and blood vessels in the Western understanding of organ systems. It needs to be understood that the chakras can hardly be localized in time or space. They are the gateways to other realities and levels of consciousness. Another limitation of our current theory of individualism is the belief that we are each localized to a certain axis and coordinate. Nothing could be further from the truth. We interact with each other and with other avenues of reality through these subtle energy systems. To awaken to these energy systems is to awaken to other modes of existence.

There are associated physical manifestations and mental states with each chakra as follows:

(1) Base—survival

(2) Sacral—emotions and sensuality

(3) Solar plexus—personal energy and power

(4) Heart—love and relationships

(5) Throat—communications and creativity

(6) Brow—intuition, insight, and imagination

(7) Crown—knowledge and understanding

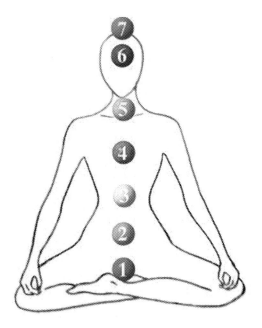

To realize that problems that manifest in our psychic and physical experiences can be explained and treated through realignment of energies is a major advancement toward healing. Quite frankly, the hubris of Western medicine has denied the existence of these immaterial yet basic energy systems. To understand that we are all a mysterious dance of energy is to take a large step toward true healing.

The other significant theory of energy healing is found in Chinese acupuncture. Vital energy, or Qi, exists throughout the body. Qi is composed of yin and yang energies that need to be in balance for optimal well-being. Internal factors causing disease arise from unbalanced emotional states: excessive anger, joy, worry, sadness, and fear. Disease can also stem from abnormal ways of eating and drinking, or from exhaustion and boredom.

External factors can also produce an imbalance of Qi flow. Wind, fire, moisture, dryness, and cold can lead to disease when present in amounts to adversely affect Qi harmony. (In our modern world Qi can be affected by numerous electromagnetic exposures, stress, poor dietary choices, inadequate sleep, and the many pressures of modern living.) These factors correlate with the solid internal organs: the liver, heart, spleen, lung, and kidney, respectively. There is a further correlation with the elements of wood, fire, earth, metal, and water. The "five element theory" has come to dominate the practice of Oriental medicine by the art of diagnosing relative emptiness, fullness, temperature, and the yin and yang energies and noting the relationship to the elements and their interrelationships of power and control. This brief summary cannot do justice to this ancient art.

When an imbalance is found, the practitioner can rebalance the person's Qi by accessing energy channels called meridians. Meridians are not lines on the body but can be pictured as rivers of energy that run through the body. For optimal health, these rivers need to be free-flowing. Each of these meridians (there are yin meridians that correlate with the solid internal organs and yang meridians that correlate with the hollow internal organs) has particular points on the skin at which these Qi channels can be accessed. Using needles, heat, or digital pressure the meridian can be manipulated to either enervate or release accumulated energies. There are fourteen major meridians and eight extra meridians that have been identified. Each meridian has points along its course that are areas where Qi flow can be accessed.

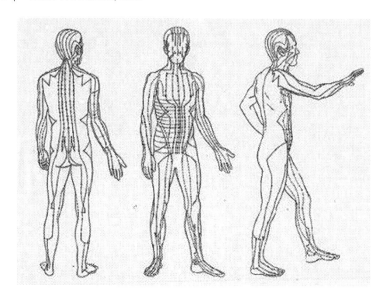

As an extension of the meridian system, the Eastern practitioners have also found correlates to organs and their dysfunctions in the ear, sole of the foot, scalp, and iris. The Oriental practitioner has also learned to examine the tongue and feel the pulse as diagnostic tools. The quality of the voice, the colors a person selects, dietary choices, and the quality of sleeping all aid in evaluating the state of Qi.

We are spirit and energy. The East has intuited this for millenia. The rationalism of the West has certainly advanced the understanding and treatment of organic disease. I have been a witness to the amazing, life-saving advances produced with the minds of our scientists and innovators. The body in crisis can now be salvaged and restored in most cases to some degree of health. The body not in crisis needs the intuition and healing techniques of the East.

Rethinking Disease

> All that we are is a result of what we have thought.
>
> The Buddha

You shall know the truth and the truth shall set you free.

Jesus of Nazareth

The supreme reality stands revealed in the consciousness of those who have conquered themselves.

The Bhagavad Gita

The great awakening that is waiting to occur is the realization that our thoughts contain much power. We are what we think. I hope that it is evident now that we are not simply a collection of chemicals and organ systems. We are a complex array of energies constantly interacting within our own bodies and with the energy systems that surround us. The quality of our inner lives and our subsequent energies determine our state of health.

An important distinction needs to be made. As I have stated, the success of modern medicine lies in its ability to treat with great success organ systems in crisis. Indeed, this is the foundation of Western medicine. These are the textbooks I studied in medical school. This has been the foundation of my professional career. Medicines and surgical procedures have been developed that save lives. The skills and knowledge of its practitioners should be utilized when one's body is potentially in a crisis state. If the sudden onset of pain, confusion, fever, trouble breathing, weakness, vomiting, bleeding, or any major trauma occurs, then you should consider seeking immediate help from a practitioner of Western medicine who has at his disposal the tools with which we diagnose and treat life-threatening illness. We may not be able to diagnose the exact cause of illness, but treatment can be procured that reverses or cures the disease process.

I contend that the weakness of Western medicine is the failure to offer appropriate treatment options to those suffering from chronic illness or who have symptoms not able to be definitively diagnosed by modern techniques. In our excitement to use science to solve problems we have failed to step back to realize our limits. Much harm is now being done to patients through the use of drug, surgery, and radiation therapies. Every day at work I see patients who are expecting a diagnosis and a curative treatment for symptoms and diseases that are not definable by Western medicine. Millions of dollars, countless hours, unnecessary radiation administration, and needless pharmaceuticals are used to appease our patients who do not have identifiable disease in the body. It is time for allopathic medicine practitioners to embrace other understandings of disease so that they can help their patients, not deceive them. Symptoms not explained through the use of modern diagnostics can be managed by expanding our definitions of disease.

All disease begins in the immaterial realm. We are mind, body and spirit. The missing link in our understanding of disease is the realization that energies are accosting our bodies from within and without at all times. To acquire health and healing we must learn to manage these energies.

Granted, there are energies that affect us that we can do little to control. Electronic media, environmental pollutants, manufactured plastics, and potential food contaminants are all part of our world and most certainly cause an appreciable accumulation of detriment to our bodies. Short of leaving the planet, these exposures will be difficult to completely contain or eradicate. Certainly there are measures to take to limit these exposures. Hopefully, our society will become more vigilant in becoming more ecologically protective and proactive. Individually, there are ways to control the effect these external energies have on our bodies. The foods we eat contain contaminants and additives that are potentially harmful. One can purify the air in one's local environment, decrease contaminants with frequent hand-washing, and limit exposures to electromagnetic radiations. There are options available to limit these exposures; however, significant decreases depend upon political and societal movements for change.

What we can control are the energies we are exposed to through our own actions, thoughts, words, emotions, and relationships. This has been the insight of the great spiritual leaders in history and has been lost amidst the onslaught of scientism. Our inner lives—thoughts, emotions, feelings, and desires—are responsible for energies that, if not appropriately balanced, can lead to bodily disease. These are the energies we need to learn to manage.

What exactly is this freedom that Jesus and the other great teachers refer to? These words of Jesus are often quoted: the truth shall set you free. What is this truth, and what exactly is this freedom? Furthermore, is this freedom related to health? I maintain that there is a deep unity in these spiritual teachings with a healthy mind, body, and spirit. Jesus talks about freedom from sin; Buddha teaches freedom from suffering; Krishna reveals the illusion of the individual self; Lao-Tzu contends that wisdom lies in unknowing. Are all of these teachings pointing to the same center?

When Jesus speaks of sin he is referring to mistakes in thinking that lead to wrong action. This is the essence of his teaching in the "Sermon on the Mount" in Matthew's Gospel. We act improperly because we think improperly. Repent simply means to rethink. The sinful act begins in the mind. Pride, anger, lust, greed, and envy are powerful emotions. When engaged by the mind the thought begins an avalanche of energy. On a physiologic level these emotions cause the release of biochemicals that lead to a much higher energy state in the individual. In the immaterial realm these energies can be harbored in the body, eventually leading to an unnatural, unbalanced energy state. These states are the precursors of disease.

Capture in your mind an episode of anger. What happens? The heart quickens, the blood pressure rises, you become agitated, and you perspire. These are all energies brought about by a thought. What if you frequent an unhealthy mental state such as is seen in anxiety, stress, and worry? There is a continuous level of energy release. If these energies are not appropriately managed, then they are retained in the body. Over time these energies accumulate in organ systems to cause disease. We can learn how to release and balance these energies. Most important, we can learn how to control and ultimately change our thinking.

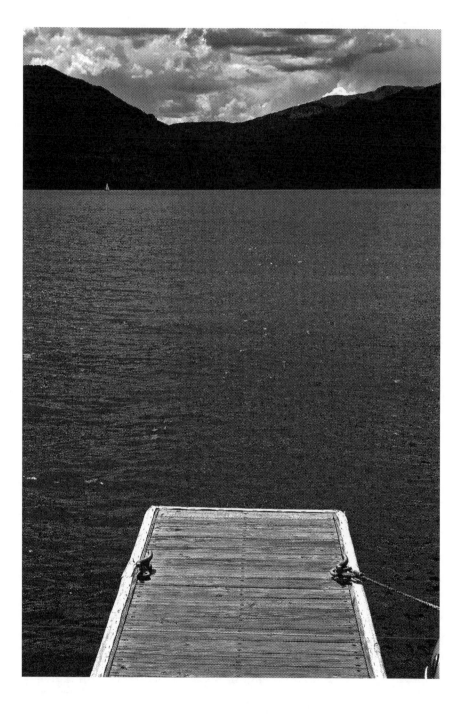

Part IV: Healing: Esoteric and Exoteric

But we have this treasure in earthen vessels to show that the transcendent power belongs to God and not to us.

Paul of Tarsus, II Cor. 4:15

What you are looking for is what is looking.

Francis of Assisi

Choose the path that leads to Nirvana.

Buddha

The essence of healthy living is to purify our patterns of living. Our thoughts, actions, diet, and habits need to be reexamined. We need collectively and individually to look beneath the surfaces of the physical world of appearances to seek ultimate truths. It is not an easy journey. The ego will fight and kick the whole way. The collective and individual self-definitions will attempt to maintain their superiority, their illusions. There will be dark places. But these spaces can be conquered with a solid foundation. That foundation is belief in a higher truth. The Kingdom of Heaven that lies within is the path Jesus directs us toward. It is the only path to healing. (Again, the Buddhist, Hindi, Taoist, Sufi, and Kabbalist mystics all describe the same journey. The name is not important. It is the same state of existence that transcends religions.)

There are healers who can assist in one's health journey, but not without the necessary inner path being confronted and engaged.

Remember where we've been. Societies' assumptions regarding the individual are found wanting. Our modern cultures' presumption of physical appearances manifesting ultimate reality has been discounted. Mind and spirit interact in mysterious ways to affect bodily function. Thoughts have energy. Spirit can be accessed to manage energy flow.

The soul of man hungers for this spiritual trek. My readings and meditations have revealed and inspired a different paradigm for health, concepts that are not new and desperately need to be rediscovered by our stressed, anxious, and distracted modern world. By what means can one balance, harness, and discover these roads to recovery?

Two Paths: Exoteric and Esoteric

There exist strategies for healing that are eternal. These the individual must pursue. There are teachers that can aid and abet one's inner journey, but the journey is ultimately one of individual intent.

I propose the following five-tiered plan for inner healing:

1. Seek God through a daily routine of contemplative prayer (meditation).

2. Commit to prolonged periods of silence and solitude.

3. Devote significant time to selfless service.

4. Purify the thought life.

5. Discipline the body in habits of eating and exercise.

A dedicated pursuit of these patterns of living I believe will result in inner healing over time.

I propose seeking the help of healers skilled in the following disciplines:

1. Acupuncture

2. Reiki

3. Chiropractic/osteopathic manipulations

4. Emotional Release Therapy/chakra manipulators

5. Massage therapy

6. Psychotherapy

A pursuit of healthier living from these practices coupled with a commitment to inner healing I believe to be an excellent foundation for a healthier life. The intended purpose of all of these practices is meant to balance, access, release, and optimize energies that could lead to disease.

Let us explore these pathways in more detail.

Esoteric Healing

(1) Quest for the Divine

There is a crisis in modern medicine. It has little to do with payer systems, technology, utilization, or access. It has everything to do with the removal of God from the arena of health care. All the medicines and technologies that our modern medicine can offer do nothing to fulfill the need of every human, the need for a spiritual quest. Even the mention of the Divine is inadequate in words. The One, the Light, YHWH, the Source, Abba, the I AM, and Brahman are all impoverished words to describe what we are pursuing. For in using language we put images in our mind's eye that limit the ultimate reality. God may or may not be anthropomorphic, but to place a certain image of the Divine reality in our mind's eye will diminish what we are seeking. We are seeking peace, light, compassion, forgiveness, and indescribable joy— "Peace that surpasses understanding," as the apostle Paul describes the experience in his letter to the church at Philippi. Left to its own devices the ego will seek distraction, despair, and disease in a futile attempt to fill the void inside. What we are seeking is timeless, formless, and uncreated.

It is time to rid ourselves of the notion that the Divine is somehow far removed from us humans, sitting in judgment, patriarchal and severe. God is within and without. God is the essence, consciousness, the "still point of the turning world," to use Eliot's terminology. It is this source from which we came, and it is to this source that we will return. This is the mystery, and it cannot be shrouded in dogma or religion. Without this as our central earthly aim our earthly lives will be incomplete, unfulfilled. This is a space in all of our lives that can be filled by no other and ironically is there all the time. It is for us to awaken to the Presence.

How does one begin this quest? First we must realize that this deep, essential need exists. Becoming aware of the inadequacy of individualism and materialism as foundational worldviews is a start. Then it is time to search for a mentor, fellow travelers. This leads us back to the great teachers: Jesus, Buddha, Krishna, Lao-Tzu, and their followers. Their message to seekers is the same: one seeks God in prayer.

This is a most difficult decision to make and subsequent journey to undertake. The ego, the mind, will denounce this pursuit as false, for it is the temporal, earthly things for which it yearns. This is the essence of the spiritual battle. To tame and to purify the mind is the nature of the spiritual quest. It is the hardest undertaking a person can pursue. It is not just a battle in one's lifetime; it is *the* battle in life. This is the battlefront of spiritual warfare. It can only be conquered through prayer, and it is hard work. The battle that ensues is fierce. The mind and our bodies seek power, pleasure, comfort, possessions, and constant distraction. These things define us to the world and give to us our sense of self. To realize that this sense of self is false is the most important insight on the journey to healing.

There is only one Consciousness, one Light. All religious study leads to this conclusion. The minds of each of the billions of people in the world attest to their individuality. To protect an image of separateness is a priority for the ego. It is the root cause of all major conflicts in the world's history. Our free-market capitalism thrives on this illusion, every person having different tastes and desires all enslaved by the mind to make itself unique. That is why we can never be filled in the empty pursuit of earthly desires. We are only made complete by seeking the One, the Source, the Light. This is our home, our true life, and our ultimate reality. To seek this enlightenment is the one true journey of the soul.

The journey from the self, the mind, the ego to the one true God is made in deep contemplative prayer. How does one pray? This seems a simple pursuit and indeed gets little attention in the preaching of modern organized religions. Perhaps because the purpose of organized religion is membership, not enlightenment. We say prayers at night before we go to bed and maybe briefly at times during the day; certainly in times of crisis we take comfort in the perceived presence of the Divine. Friends may ask for prayers, and we may want some beneficence from the Divine, so we will make requests. Certainly, worship and adoration are a vital part of personal and community prayer.

This is all well and good and may be of some benefit, but is not the kind of prayer that leads to wellness or any kind of direct communion with God. There may be a brief moment of elation, transcendence, especially during times of worship. But these are emotional responses without the depth needed for Divine communion. We need to pray with all our heart, mind, soul, and strength. We need to go into a dark room and shut the door and pray. Indeed, the door is narrow on the road that leads to enlightenment. And there are no shortcuts.

The saints of the church provide much-needed direction regarding this journey. Perhaps the evangelical tradition has had similar instructors—I have not found them to be as insightful. By minimizing the faith experience in Christ to a simple proclamation of belief, the evangelical Protestant tradition has subsequently denied believers of the experience of the Christ-consciousness. John of the Cross and Theresa of Avila both describe the journey to Light as one of detachment and darkness. The worldly self must completely dissolve in order to be in accordance with the Divine will. Purification occurs through an active denial of excessive worldly pleasures and desires but ultimately occurs passively as we are changed during the "dark night," as St. John of the Cross names it. We often will feel quite alone as our wills and characters are patterned after the will of God. The only way to succeed is to be absorbed in times of deep prayer and meditation.

Once an awareness of the battle can be visualized by the mind's eye, it is time to begin habits that foster this Divine action to proceed successfully. This cannot be overemphasized. At some point one must leap into the water. Reading, studying, and intellectualizing the journey will not take one to the depth required to instill change and healing. One must learn to pray.

Water is a prominent theme in the Gospels. Jesus calms the storms on the sea. Jesus walks on water. Jesus tells Nicodemus that one must be born of water. Jesus turns water into wine. The mind is a rushing torrent of unending chatter. It is the river that needs to be quieted if the prayer would find communion with the Divine. It is an illuminating experience to watch one's thoughts for a short while or to try to focus on one thing for any length of time. The mind will constantly flow with its diversions, ideas, and chatter. Where *do* thoughts arise?

The great teachers and mystics in the spiritual traditions offer several foundations for effective prayer. Periods of meditation always begin with the breath. The importance of learning appropriate breathing cannot be overemphasized. It is the root of healing. This is stressed in all healing traditions. Any study of yoga is centered upon control of the breath. Slow, deep breaths balance and control the flow of energy through the body and mind.

Reserve a time during the day when you will be assured an extended period of silence without interruption. Sit in a comfortable position in a comfortable chair. Your back should be supported, but the head should be held erect. Take a slow, deep breath through the nose. Feel it, pull it down into the abdomen, through the diaphragm. This is a deep, full breath that one should feel filling the chest and torso as energy rises and expands. The gateway through one's energy potential can be reached, explored, and maximized. Hold the breath for several seconds. What do you feel? There is an accumulation of energy that should fill the senses and lead to a feeling of calm and peace. Then slowly release the breath through the mouth. Continue to breathe in this manner for several minutes.

While breathing deeply, occupy your mind with a repetitive, meaningful spiritual saying. It is easy to time the mental repetition of the words with the breath. In the Eastern traditions this is called a mantra. Through the practice of using a mantra, the mind can be stilled and calmed and the storm quieted. In the Jesus tradition, several sayings have been proven to be centering:

1. The Jesus Prayer: "Lord Jesus Christ, Son of God, have mercy on me."

2. The Lord's Prayer: "Our Father, who art in Heaven, hallowed be thy name. Thy Kingdom come, thy will be done, on earth as it is in Heaven. Give us today our daily bread. Forgive us our sins as we forgive those who sin against us. Lead us not into temptation. Deliver us from evil. For thine is the Kingdom, and the Power, and the Glory, forever and ever. Amen."

3. Maranatha (Come, O Lord)

4. My God and my All

5. The Beatitudes (Matt. 5:1–10)

6. The 23rd Psalm

In the Eastern tradition these mantra have been used:

1. A—OM (the sound of the universe)

2. Om mani padme hom (very loosely translated as "Behold! The jewel in the lotus!" the path to perfection in Buddhism)

The prayer chooses a particular mantra and enters a period of meditation by repeating the mantra over and over, the words conforming to the pattern of breathing. It is a life-changing experience to calm the mind and become aware of the fullness of life that lies beneath. One should concentrate more and more on the periods between thoughts. What is present at those times? It cannot be adequately described to the novice or uninitiated. As the mind acquires the habit, the pattern of saying a particular mantra over and over then can be accessed at times of duress to give peace and calm in order to assuage and manage the negative energies of stress, fear, anxiety, and worry. The words of the mantra will spontaneously arise to calm the storm. But one has to commit to training the mind to achieve this end result.

The goal is to be in a state of centering; again, a state that is hard to describe. I think of it as being on a small island, calm and serene, in the middle of a rushing stream. I watch the water flow by just as I watch my thoughts flow by. To be centered is to be in a state of unity, detached, witnessing the sights and sounds that your senses bring to you. There is recognition of the world of the senses, but one is detached from it.

What happens next? In deep meditation you are no longer in the realm of conscious thought. When your mind is distracted, cleared, and centered by this mantra while controlled breathing is balancing energies, you gradually experience the consciousness of the Divine. Human language will always be unsatisfactory to describe this world. What happens is what happens. The pray-er will be changed. The outer world of the senses and desires will be increasingly false, and the inner world will become more real. The illusory nature of our bodies, senses, and feelings becomes apparent. What was once important will be increasingly less so. The danger now lies in not wanting to reenter the physical world. Jesus teaches clearly that we must seek and find enlightenment so that we can be lights unto others. Remember, it is no longer the individual will that determines action. If we are enlightened by God's light we cannot remain cloistered. I find the prayer of St. Francis to encapsulate the new vision:

> O Lord, make me an instrument of your peace.
> Where there is hatred, let me sow love,
> Where there is injury, pardon,

Where there is darkness, light,
Where there is despair, hope,
Where there is doubt, faith,
Where there is sadness, joy.

O Divine Master, let me not so much seek to be consoled as to console,
To be understood, as to understand,
To be loved as to love.
For it is in giving that we receive,
It is in pardoning that we are pardoned,
It is in dying to self that we are born into eternal life.
Amen.

There is no more succinct description of the road to healing the human soul.

How do these practices and themes relate to healing? If one allows the priorities of the self to reign, then one will succumb to the vagaries of desire. Attachments to worldly pursuits will control one's life. The pursuit of pleasure, power, pride, and possessions will be the individual's purpose. These pursuits will lead in all cases ultimately to despair, disappointment, and anxiety. These emotional states will lead to energies that will need to be harbored somewhere depending on the individual.

Remember my emergency room patients: no organic pathologies could be determined with the tools of modern medicine. Migraines, abdominal and chest pains, and neurological symptoms, to name the most common bodily manifestations, are a result of these imbalanced energies. To become aware of inappropriate pursuits leads one to the awareness of higher purposes to living. To extinguish and control the stormy desires of the outer self, the outer mind will lead one to the peace and healing found in the center: Divine communion.

I can speak of the practice of contemplative prayer in the Christian tradition because that is the path that I have pursued and also because I have been called to believe in the paschal mystery and the living

Christ through the Holy Spirit. By no means does this discount the experiences of those practicing meditation in the Hindu, Buddhist, Sufi, or the Kabbalist traditions. As I have stated earlier, I believe strongly that the paths are parallel if not identical. It seems likely to me that Krishna achieved the same transcendent consciousness that Jesus had attained. I suspect that the Buddhist concept of Nirvana is very much the same as the Kingdom of Heaven of which Jesus speaks. The Sufi poet Rumi writes of a path that parallels the Christian mystics' journey. In the Kabbalist tradition one journeys toward a unity as well. I do not know. Not commenting on these non-Christian pathways by no means diminishes their validity as pathways to Truth. A traveler cannot describe paths he has not traversed.

(2) Seeking Silence and Solitude

The omnipresence of the mass media is poisoning the modern mind. We as a culture are distracted and diffused by the constant influx of stimuli. It is theorized that the constant deluge of electromagnetic radiation is cumulatively detrimental to one's health. Even more destructive is the occupation of our minds with detritus. Perhaps the first step on the journey to enlightenment is to turn off the television, give away the iPod, limit movie viewing, and say no to the emptiness of our culture's current art forms. It is intriguing to me to witness the immense cultural popularity of Internet-based entertainments and the rise of its pseudo-communities. Leisure time is now consumed by Internet-based activities. At least one should not make them a priority of daily living.

Every great spiritual teacher has recognized the importance of silence in questing for peace. Committing to times of solitude allows escape from the noise and clutter of daily living. An awareness of the inner self can only occur when the outer mind is not distracted. This constant need for entertainment and distraction is really the modern addiction. The mind readily takes advantage of this torrent of stimuli. It is indeed upon what the mind thrives! We cater to its whims. When called by his disciples, Jesus awakened to calm the storm. We can calm the mind's storm by first of all limiting its external fuel.

To begin, a short period of each day can be reserved for quiet; maybe early morning or late evening. No TV, radio, or any distractions. Select a favorite chair or room where you are comfortable and distractions will be at a minimum. This is amazingly difficult for the mind to agree to! If the initial opposition can be thwarted, then you will find yourself craving these periods of quiet. Begin a routine of breathing, scripture reading, perhaps yoga, as a prelude to deep prayer/meditation. This will become a cornerstone to premium health if this practice is maintained.

By disengaging from the hectic pace of modern life and the worry and anxiety that is involved with daily living, one can escape from selfish attachment. It is in silence that the riches of meditation can be achieved. It is in solitude that the illusion of the self can be fully realized. This is initiated with a conscious awareness of the need to slow down. If there is a commitment to periods of silence and solitude, then it is much easier to realize and achieve a slower pace of life.

Krishna has these words of wisdom from the Gita:

> Select a clean spot, neither too high nor too low, and seat yourself firmly on a cloth. Then, once seated, strive to still your thoughts. Make your mind one-pointed in meditation, and your heart will be purified. Hold your head, body, and neck firmly in a straight line, and keep your eyes from wandering. With all fears dissolved in the peace of the Self and all desires dedicated to Brahman, controlling the mind and fixing it on me, sit in meditation with me as your only goal.

This summarizes the aim of the spiritual aspirant. This is the path to true healing of the spirit. It is pursued in silence and solitude. For the Christ-follower it may be difficult to read about the Self, Brahman, Krishna, Nirvana, and other terms used by the Eastern mystic. Do not be put off. Escape from the patterning of your mind that you have learned. Unlearn your notions of exclusivity. The Light is indivisible by sects or religion. Dogma has distracted the mind from the true path. "If you want to become full, let yourself become empty," says the Tao.

(3) Selfless Service

The great paradox of true spiritual wisdom is that we most fully become ourselves when we give ourselves away. The first step is in gaining the insight that life is not about seeking one's individual pleasure, worldly successes, possessions, and control. A commitment to prayer, spiritual readings, and times of solitude will provide this necessary insight. The next step is to seek and to serve the inner Light.

All sincere efforts to serve others begin at home. I see the path to selfless service as a series of concentric circles. One starts in the service of the Divine, and then one learns to serve those at home, then friends and one's immediate community, then the workplace, and then extending outward. To what end or means do we serve? As we peel away the layers of our selfishness our light can shine for others.

People need many things. There are the physical requirements of shelter, food, hygiene, comfort; the emotional pain of the lonely, ill, depressed, and despairing demands a keen development of awareness; the closed intellectualism of the minds in the wake of individualism and materialism need to be opened with an attitude of gentle kindness to the beauty and peace of the One; and finally there is an awareness of the deep unity that exists in the religious pursuits of mankind to move away from this culture of destruction that religious exclusiveness fosters.

There has been a commitment to service in the global arena by the Western religious traditions that has been a blessing to the world, from affluent societies to those who are oppressed. This is all well and good. However, this global outreach cannot be at the expense of these circles of service. One cannot begin to serve without addressing the relentless pursuit of the Divine Light, the needs of one's immediate family and community, and one's workplace. Each of our individual ministries begins at home. We cannot climb the mountain without before we conquer the mountain within. We cannot change the world if we do not change ourselves first.

Become aware. Learn to live completely in the moment. What do those around us need? Where is their pain? How can we help? Perhaps all a loved one needs is a caring concern, attentive listening, a commitment to their welfare. The greatest gift we can give is our time. If one minimizes the distractions in one's thought life, there will be ample time for selfless service.

There are many ways to give of one's self. Time, listening, gifts of various types, physical tasks, phone calls, cooking, cleaning—the types of service are endless. What is needed is a deep understanding that we are here for a higher purpose. To shift one's focus from the self to others is one of life's greatest achievements. As we become closer to God it becomes easier to enter into selfless service.

(4) Changing Our Minds

Detachment, humility, and prayer are the cornerstones upon which a spiritual life is built. These attributes encapsulate the teachings of the masters. We are attached to many things in this earthly existence. Think about the ways in which you might describe yourself to others. Career, spouse, family, hometown, education, and interests are all attachments. Even spiritual pursuits can evolve into an attachment. Illnesses can become attachments. All of these describe the outer mind. Granted, all are an essential component of the human experience, but they do not define who one is or what one should be doing. To continue to be defined in these terms limits the awareness and prohibits access to higher states of consciousness. It is fine to enjoy travel or football, but we must stop being attached to these activities.

One of the great parables in the Gospels relates to Jesus and the rich man. The man comes to Jesus asking for wisdom. Jesus responds by telling him to give away his possessions. The rich man cannot do this; he is too attached to them. Subsequently, he is unable to attain higher levels of awareness, "eternal life." How difficult! Each of us has spent a lifetime acquiring experiences that define us. The message is clear that these definitions limit us.

The great teachers dedicate a significant portion of their teachings to instructing the seeker on the importance of changing one's thinking. Repentance, after all, is nothing more than asking the aspirant to change his mind, the patterns of thinking. In the first Gospel to be written, the Gospel of Mark, Jesus calls for two actions from the seeker: repentance and hearing (the Good News). What is the Good News? The Good News is the realization that we can be free from the attachments and the illusions that enslave our minds. This is achieved through a realization of the Christ-consciousness through the Holy Spirit that moves around and through us. The Sermon on the Mount in Matthew's Gospel is a diatribe on the dangers of improper thinking and how to rectify them. Krishna devotes much of his teaching in the Gita to the misunderstanding of our minds regarding who we are and what we should be doing. The Tao attempts to instruct the aspirant on the proper thinking that is required to reach the source. We are what we have thought is the Buddha's teaching.

The hardest attachments to release are emotional ones. So much of our thought lives is given to ruminations on our pain. Anger, fear, envy, greed, pride, and lust are thoughts that consume the mind. How difficult to see past the illusion. The ego is desperate in its attempts to elevate itself above other egos. How much of life is spent in empty pursuits! The mind is consumed by past hurts and regrets and is distraught over what may or may not occur in the future. The present, the moment is all.

The greatest power in the world is forgiveness. This should give us pause. Forgive yourself for not being attractive or powerful enough; forgive others for past wrongs, real or perceived. "You will know the truth and the truth will set you free," says Jesus. Is this the truth? We are not slaves to our sin, our thoughts and actions that are removed from the Divine will. How much healing would occur if the practice of forgiveness were incorporated daily into our lives?

The Lord's Prayer commands that we forgive others' sins while we are asking forgiveness from God. There is no *quid pro quo*. The forgiveness of others precedes or is at least simultaneous to the forgiveness we receive from the Father. Let us accept imperfections in ourselves and in others. As the father rushes to embrace the prodigal son, so we should rush to forgive those who have injured us. This may be the most important recommendation for healing that I know.

Initiate habits that result in purification of the thought life: reading scripture, mantra repetition, minimizing external media distractions, minimizing multi-tasking, and practicing mindfulness. Mindfulness is an Eastern concept that is very important—learning to focus the mind on the task at hand, whether that be listening to a friend or performing your work. Our minds rush to focus on the future, lingering on things that may or may not happen. The mind also has learned from the past, has been trained by the past so that much of its time is spent rehashing past events or patterning present or future events on past experiences. Complete attention given to the present is a very challenging yet essential habit for the modern mind. There are so many distractions to confront. Our minds thrive and seek these distractions. Remember the words of Jesus to his disciples on the boat: "Peace! Be still!"

Avoid situations that lead to unwanted distraction. Avoid situations that lead to sin. Limit contacts with friends and colleagues who are discouraging and impure. Seek activities that increase spirituality and truth. Often we find ourselves wallowing in debauchery, and our attachment to it prohibits release. Become aware of your attachments. Practice prayer.

As we move along this path of purity, there will still be worldly temptations and situations with people or places that can lead one to return to past habits of thought and action. When one is ensconced in impurity, the mind needs to turn to prayer. The great power that lies within needs to be recognized. The ego's attachment to impure thoughts and actions will gradually diminish as one focuses on the purity of the inner life. If the mind strays to thoughts of lust, envy, greed, or anger, allow yourself to feel the emotional state. Do not suppress it, but gradually bring the mind into prayer through use of the mantra and with meditative breathing. This is indeed a powerful tool. For emotions will not disappear; they do need to be removed from their position of power. Over time, these strong emotions can be easily controlled and the mind redirected. This is not an easy battle! It may indeed be the only battle. To control the mind's torrent of emotion may be life's greatest battle. The ego is a worthy opponent.

To be detached from things does not mean they should not be enjoyed. The key point is to not focus on a personal need for the thing that is enjoyed. Pleasure enjoyed with the appropriate gratitude reflects the beneficence of the Divine. Much pain is caused through the inappropriate expression of sexual desire. What a tangled, confusing mess our current culture finds itself in regarding appropriate sexual behavior. Our culture of desire has fostered insatiable sexual lust. What amount of unhappiness occurs is immeasurable. In reading the masters of spiritual discernment, the unspoken consensus is for a cessation of sexual desire leading to an optimization of happiness.

Humility results from the acquisition of detachment and the proliferation of prayer. Jesus talks of accepting the children and becoming as a child. Both are severe expressions of humility. Do not allow the ego to deceive! There is a deep unity behind the illusion of the ego. Free yourself.

(5) Proper Maintenance

Nutritional indiscretion and fitness complacency are the two greatest health problems facing the West today. We are killing ourselves through gluttony and sloth. The battleground is the will. Whose will has control? As we move closer to the Divine will through the aforementioned practices, it is hoped that an awareness will emerge that we have a responsibility to maintain this body with which we have been gifted. The substances we ingest matter; they are the building blocks of our physical structures. Proper exercise is beneficial for balancing energies and keeping our organ systems conditioned.

As with other impurities of thought, one needs to focus on the desires of the ego balanced in the light of healthful habits. Fast foods, chips, soft drinks, and processed foods taste good. They are readily accessible, relatively inexpensive, and aggressively marketed. It takes awareness, an alternative dietary plan, and a commitment to healthy eating to win this battle. Again, the mind can be conditioned through prayer and meditation to resist the ubiquitous societal plea to engage the desires of the ego. Healthy dietary plans are readily available.

Vegetarian lifestyles are easily supportable in this era of unnatural, cruel livestock management. That is an individual choice. Certainly, meat should be ingested in moderation. The Buddhist avers that the energies of the ingested substance will be absorbed. I agree. If livestock or fish have spent a life being prepared for slaughter in unnatural living conditions it is easy to surmise the turmoil present at some level in the animal psyche. This would result in retained negative energies in its tissue. Where do these energies go?

Moderation in eating, proper choices, and a control of desire for unhealthy foods need to be at the center of a dietary plan. Eating good food is one of the great pleasures in life. Sharing a communal meal is a necessary and beneficial practice. It needs to be done mindfully. One should incorporate a slowness in eating, chewing food completely before swallowing, eating with an attitude of thanksgiving for the preparer and gatherer of the meal and the ability to enjoy good food.

What should one eat? What should one avoid? It is common sense that many of today's foods are not healthy. Processed foods, fast foods, alcohol, simple sugars, and enriched flours should be avoided. Naturally colorful foods are good for you! Fruits, vegetables, whole grains, nuts, coconut oil, and nonmeat protein sources are all excellent choices. In particular, excellent dietary choices include blueberries, tomatoes, sweet potatoes, walnuts and almonds, yogurt, black beans, avocadoes, pomegranates, and numerous fiber-laden food sources. Dairy should be consumed from organic producers and ingested sparingly. Meats if eaten should be from free-range sources. Eggs are excellent sources of protein but should be from organic suppliers.

I find it easy to make an argument for vegetarian living, but my conditioned dietary responses make vegetarianism an ongoing struggle. Again, it is beyond the scope of this book to provide a complete regimen for healthy eating. These sources are readily available in the marketplace. It is my intent to create awareness for the need of a healthier lifestyle.

It is a modern challenge to find foods that are not contaminated by a variety of additives. Pesticides, antibiotics, heavy metals, bacteria, and viruses, to name a few of the known contaminants, have invaded our food supply. Most of these are anthropogenic, introduced in the production of food to increase supply to our culture of insatiable appetites. Let the buyer/consumer beware! Our most available and inexpensive foods are slowly killing us. Cancer rates increase annually, and diabetes, hypertension, kidney disease, and heart disease are likely either directly or indirectly attributable to these additives. Obesity is an epidemic in our gluttonous society. The battle is fought with the mind, the will. The craving for food is one of mankind's deepest urges. Food serves many purposes. Stress appeasement, aphrodisiac, community ritual, worship, and healing are all purposes for which food plays a central role. It is for us to readdress our current misuses of food in our pleasure-centered culture.

The purification of what we eat, breathe, and touch is a major modern challenge. Our culture has contaminated our air and soil with numerous contaminants. Disease can be easily transmitted by touch or inhalation. Several steps can minimize these risks, such as frequent hand-washing, air purification through filtering or opening windows, minimizing the use of plastics, and vacuuming frequently.

An overlooked component of proper maintenance is adequate sleep. My patients are overworked, overstressed, and sleep-deprived. Much of our insomnia can be fixed through behavior modification: decreasing caffeine, cigarette, alcohol, and junk food consumption; turning off the television and limiting other modern media distractions; avoiding late-night eating; and improving time-management skills. A busy, stimulated mind will be difficult to quiet. Develop a pattern of evening prayer or meditation so that the torrent of thought can be tamed and rest will come more readily.

The other part of maintaining a healthy lifestyle is fighting sloth. Exercise is an integral component of healing. Most of us can relate to the seeming paradox of having a surge of energy during and after exercising when beforehand there was a feeling of fatigue and listlessness. Moving our bodies energizes us! It is now becoming apparent that strenuous, painful regimens are not needed and may indeed be harmful. Brisk walking for thirty minutes a day is a good place to start. Several times a week or preferably on a daily basis a period of vigorous walking will produce long-lasting health benefits. Practicing the Eastern arts of yoga or Qi Gong is an excellent way to produce and maintain balanced energy states.

Again, the ego will fight back. That objects at rest tend to remain at rest is a principle of Newtonian macrophysics. The ego indulges itself in pleasures. It will always be easier to eat rich, unhealthy foods requiring minimal preparation, to remain distracted by modern entertainments, to accept the status quo. It takes a focused, determined will established in meditation and a realigned sense of self to overcome.

Exoteric Healing

Throughout the ages healers of all cultures have known of techniques that access, cleanse, and balance the energies that lead to disease. The hubris of modern scientism denounces these practices. It is time to acknowledge the acquired wisdom of the collective human experience to maximize healing therapies. We need the discernment of wise medical professionals to direct patients into the hands of appropriate healers. There certainly are times to utilize modern diagnostics, pharmacotherapies, and surgical techniques. There are also times to admit that alternative, traditional treatment options exist and are beneficial. These involve treatments affecting the latent or imbalanced human energy systems.

(1) Chiropractic manipulation

Literally "done by hand," chiropractic manipulation has been around for a relatively short amount of time. Developed in the late 1800s when a healer cured a man of deafness through spinal manipulation, chiropractics now is a popular and effective healing technique. Denounced and disparaged by modern allopathic physicians, it nonetheless has helped people recover from a variety of medical ailments and symptoms. Few of these can be experimentally studied through the use of the scientific method. Why does chiropractic manipulation relieve back pain, cold symptoms, and gastrointestinal disorders? Modern medicine has no answer to these queries; therefore, it is chided as a form of quackery. Perhaps the healing occurs through the balance of energies, a form of energy realignment.

The spine harbors and bisects the major energy channels of the body. Chiropractic theory maintains that there are displacements of vertebrae that, when adjusted, result in symptom relief and healing. I maintain that this is simply a form of chakra energy adjustment: a form of massage therapy, if you will. The two central autonomic nervous system pathways are situated adjacent to the spinal cord. Likewise, the acupuncturist utilizes meridians adjacent to the spinal column. Why should it seem unusual for the chiropractor to induce healing by "adjusting" the spine?

Osteopathic manipulation treats presumed spinal imbalances in a similar fashion, either through gentle manipulation or by using a technique of brisk, localized pressure at an affected joint. Regardless, people feel better, and that cannot be denied. The benefits of direct touch in human energy systems cannot be underestimated.

(2) Acupuncture

To enter into a brief synopsis of this ancient Chinese healing practice is to do it a great disservice. This ancient art has been practiced in the East for more than two thousand years. It has just recently been introduced to the West. The knowledge and experience that is required is extensive and is coupled with an acute sense of observation, intuition, and listening.

The practice is based on the balancing of energies through the access of energy pathways called meridians. These lines of energies are well described in acupuncture literature. Points along these lines can be penetrated using needles to release or increase energies in the meridian based upon the clinician's diagnosis of yin or yang energy condition. These acupuncture points could also be stimulated or suppressed by digital pressure, laser, heating lamps, cupping, or by igniting the Chinese herb *moxa* and placing it over a point.

In addition, the pulses are felt and aid in diagnosis based on their relative strength and rhythm. The tongue and the eyes also serve as gateways for the practitioner to sense the patient's energies. The timing of symptoms is correlated with particular organ activities, again to give a clue as to which energies need rebalancing.

Much research has demonstrated the efficacy of acupuncture therapies. Respiratory and neurological conditions are quite susceptible to these treatments. Heart disease, mental disease, and nausea have also been treated successfully. Let us open our minds to these ancient treatment options.

(3) Massage therapies

Human touch can heal. In the West we suffer from "touch-deficiency." Our media markets are so focused on the power of sexuality to incite consumer desires that we have lost the ability to appreciate the beauty and sensitivities involved in nonsexual touch. What a deep loss for the human experience. If spouses would focus their attentions on nonsexual touch I imagine marital disharmony would dramatically decrease. The powerful healing that comes through touch is the basis for the effectiveness of massage.

Massage helps relieve anxiety, depression, musculoskeletal disorders, and potentially many other ailments. Pressure can be applied along acupuncture meridians, major muscle groups, joints, the spine, and in reflexology, along points on the soles that correlate with major organ groups. There are traditions of massage in the East that have been practiced for centuries. I would again maintain that the practitioner is doing nothing more than rebalancing misdirected energies.

(4) Reiki

Japanese for "universal life energy," developed by a Japanese educator in the mid-1800s, Reiki is now enjoying a loyal following. It is available to everyone. One can easily access these energies to transmit them to others. Recall the teaching of the modern quantum physicist: "all is energy." Through meditation and controlled breathing these energies can be realized through practice and recognition. The energies can be felt in the palm of one's hands; the palms actually feel hot, and the energies are directed to the individual's or the patient's affected area of concern. This is the Qi energy of the Chinese, the prana of the Indian. It is the Holy Spirit, I believe, if one honors it as such.

The practitioner will "scan" the body to gauge areas of energy depletion. The hands can be trained to feel differences in energy fields, therefore being able to sense areas of the body that need treatment. The hands can then be placed over these particular areas and energy can be "sent" through the hands to these depleted areas. The only requirement to use these energies is to become aware of them and then to nourish them through prayer, yoga, and opening chakra channels of energy.

The only spurious attribute of Reiki is the presumed need for a practitioner to be "attuned" by a Reiki master. Reiki is healing through the use of a universal energy source and is unlimited in its availability. Experienced, gifted energy healers have learned how to access certain vibrational energy states that facilitate healing energies to be transmitted to the afflicted. I am not convinced that others can be elevated to this same state of energy without advanced meditation techniques. However, in the yogic traditions and Catholic traditions mystics can elevate those around them just by being in their vicinity. This probably occurs rarely in today's world. Regardless, Reiki energies are not unique. However, a committed Reiki practitioner healing with intention is capable of transmitting and balancing dysfunctional energy systems in the body.

(5) Chakra healing

I have personally experienced healing on myself and on others through the opening or balancing of Chakra energy centers. My friend Walter Weston has developed a technique called Emotional Release Therapy that directly accesses the heart chakra. For years Walter has been helping people release unhealthy, harbored energies with remarkable results.

This therapy requires one to place a hand over the fourth chakra, the heart chakra, and the hand acts as a conduit for the release of energies. The heart chakra is thought to communicate with others and therefore is susceptible to energy depletions or enhancements relative to the impact others have upon us. To interact with others is to be vulnerable to their energies. There are people who energize us; there are people who deplete us. If one has been subject to great psychic sufferings incurred through one's own actions or the actions of others, then one needs somehow to release these energies. The central thesis of this tome lies in this very concept: harmful, mismanaged emotional states leave us with harmful, mismanaged energies. If this is not recognized then dis-ease results.

This therapy can be self-administered. Place one hand over the heart chakra. Meditate for a few moments. To release harmful, retained emotions envision a color or an object. Then feel fully the harmful emotion that has plagued you. Allow this emotion to attach to this color or object that has been visualized and visualize it flowing through the fourth chakra. As this is occurring the hand that is located over the chakra should become hot as these energies are released. It is important to fully feel the emotion so it can be released. This can be difficult in the turmoil of the mind.

A facilitator can be enlisted to help in this release. A healer can place a hand over the chakra in lieu of the patient's own hand. The same procedure is utilized. Then one centers the focus through meditation and deep breathing. This is followed by a release of toxic emotions through the heart chakra. Remember, chakras are spinning wheels of energy that are spinning into the environment around us and around others.

I believe that simply holding a hand over a chakra can result in similar healing results. During prayer, chakra energies can be balanced in the same way. This is the same principle upon which Reiki is based, except that we are focusing our energies upon the chakra channels specifically. Again, a feeling of increasing warmth in the hand and likely more diffuse sensations of energies should be experienced.

The purpose of many yoga practices is aimed at balancing chakra systems. Each yoga position is developed to move energy through one or more chakra energy fields. By an analysis of one's particular somatic dysfunction one can rebalance these energies by focusing on a particular yoga position.

Beware of the release of these toxic energies! In my work I have struggled with the appropriate release of these energies. If I absorb them, then I feel feelings of nausea, weakness, and generalized malaise. Most healers suggest periodically placing the hand used in healing into a saltwater solution to disperse the energies. This practice prevents the patient or the healer from reclaiming or from resorbing these harmful energies.

(6) Psychotherapy

It is very difficult to step outside of one's psyche and see the negative effects of long-term behaviors and beliefs. Most of these attitudes, beliefs, and resultant habits of thought and action have been learned at a young age. Unless one seeks an objective analysis true transformation will be difficult. It is hard to see one's self objectively.

An experienced psychotherapist is able to assess unhealthy behaviors and redirect a client to realize the illusory nature of these associations. At their core these behaviors are rooted in the ego and its desperate attempt to gain complete control over the individual. We must again ask the great questions to pursue a path of healing. Exactly what is an individual? Once one peels off layer after layer of ego illusion we are left with nothing except the wonderful, limitless present moment of complete awareness.

Typically, the therapist will take a client into some degree of meditation/hypnosis so that the subconscious mind can be accessed. When the subconscious is accessed, thoughts and memories will be brought to the surface so that we can identify our behaviors with past experiences. We can subsequently realize our false attachment to these learned behaviors. Quite often bodily illness will resolve when these attachments are released.

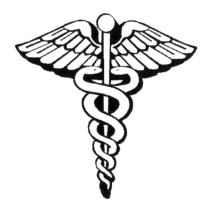 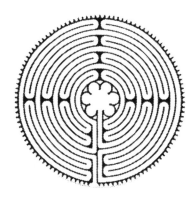

Two Symbols: One Journey

> The way up and the way down are one and the same.
>
> Heraclitus

> Our life is an apprenticeship to the truth that around
> every circle another can be drawn; that there is no end
> in nature, but every end is a beginning ... and under
> every deep a lower deep opens.
>
> R. W. Emerson

> I learned that words are no good; that words don't ever
> fit even what they are trying to say at.
>
> Addie Bundren in William Faulkner's *As I Lay Dying*

The journey to healing is an uncovering of superficial layers of the self and
our lives to reveal deeper truths and meanings. It involves a choice. The
easy choice is to remain on the surface and allow the ego to manipulate

and confuse our real selves. The hard choice is to descend into the depths where ultimately light will guide and inspire an awakening.

In the ancient world symbols were of paramount importance to communicate what words could not. Of course, our modern world is full of symbols, but unfortunately their purposes now are aimed at the ego and its consumerism potential. Symbols nonetheless move us on very deep, basic levels.

Two symbols in particular reflect the crux of this outlined path to healing: the caduceus and the labyrinth. Both of these symbols reflect the journey inward and upward that is required of the aspirant.

The caduceus comes to us from ancient mythology. It was the staff that Hermes carried with him as he worked between the gods and humankind. The staff is entwined with two serpents. As they climb skyward the staff is adorned with wings at the acme. This symbol is ubiquitous in the modern medical arena as it adorns and advertises numerous hospitals, physician offices, and ancillary service providers.

Ironically, medical providers that choose this symbol to represent their trade do so erroneously. It is actually the staff of Aeschylus that more appropriately represents the healing profession. Aeschylus was a Greek physician who reportedly would use his staff to induce healings. It is represented as a staff with one serpent entwined around it.

Most certainly the symbolism of the caduceus has been lost to the ages. It needs to be rediscovered, for its hidden meanings are profound. The staff represents the spine and the spinal cord as it ascends to the cerebral cortex. Each serpent has as its corollary a part of the autonomic nervous system— the sympathetic and parasympathetic chains that modulate subconscious bodily function. These two systems work in a delicate balance to maintain the organism's homeostasis in times of stress and calm.

The two serpents cross seven times as they ascend the staff. Seven is a significant number in the lexicon of spiritual aspirants. The Eastern mystic describes the mastery of the seven chakras to attain enlightenment. Likewise, the Western mystic (see Saint Teresa of Avila's "Seven Mansions") describes a progression of seven stages, or rooms, that one must "enter" as one progresses toward divine union in the seventh mansion or room.

As the serpents cross the seventh time the staff erupts into broad, open wings to represent the stage of enlightenment in which there is complete freedom from the physical, gravity-restricted bodily existence into the mystical unity with the Divine (the "Jewel" within the lotus). This is the realm to which saints, yogis, and Zen mystics aspire and that human language in its impoverishment cannot begin to describe.

The Eastern traditions describe a latent energy that resides in our base chakra called "kundalini." As this energy awakens, the aspirant experiences energy and power that can be utilized in various ways. This is the power and truth that every great teacher and mystic has learned to access.

The other ancient symbol is the labyrinth. Labyrinths date back to ancient times as symbolic of the spiritual journey. One traverses a pathway that winds in a diminishing centripetal direction to a focal point. Typically, the sojourner would enter into a meditative state as the labyrinth was entered, in hopes of gaining progressive states of transcendence as the center was approached. The center is representative of union with the Divine. The various stages one traverses to access the center reflects the progressive detachment the aspirant has to the ego.

The Buddhists utilize similar symbolism in their use of the mandala. These designs attain a high state of artistry as they depict as well the path of the spiritual aspirant. The main point of these symbols is to bring the seeker from outer levels of awareness to deeper meanings that become apparent as one enters the depths of psychic awareness.

The caduceus and the labyrinth summarize this journey to healing—the need to conquer the ego and its superficial desires in order to access the healing, truth, and power that exist in the love of the Divine.

The Future of Medicine

You must dance and sing and be alive in the mystery, be gracious and give thanks and let yourself go.

Van Morrison

If you saw the face of God and Love, would you change?

Tracy Chapman

I did not come to heal those who (think they) are well, but those who are sick.

Jesus of Nazareth

The practitioner in the future will be well versed in the management of energy systems. Equipped with an appreciation of modern physics, centered in the fullness of the Mystery, valuing the faith traditions of the many as they grasp the realization of the One, he or she will facilitate the realignment of unbalanced energies. Modern medical concepts involving surgery and pharmacology will be utilized conservatively. The healer will enable the patient to realize the innate healing capabilities of one's own body. Ancient and modern energy therapies will be utilized liberally. This will be done in a partnership of mutual caring and respect, fully realizing that we are in the midst of a Divine Mystery in which the aim is not the personal fulfillments of ease, comfort, pleasure, and security but rather a mystical union with the Divine so that we can be led to selflessly serve others in the eternal Light of Truth.

There will be a shifting emphasis of healing from the primary use of external sources to awakening the latent healing energies that lie within. The practitioner will focus on health instead of illness. The trinity of mind, body, and spirit in the proper maintenance of health and wellness will be paramount in treating outward manifestations of disease.

I can envision a medical education consisting of spiritual awakening, training in acupuncture, a serious pursuit for self-knowledge, and an awareness of the energy systems of the body. Let us not disparage the progress of modern medicine. Rather, it is for us to reclaim the wisdoms of the ages. We are not our own; we were bought for a price, to paraphrase the great apostle.

The patient will no longer be a passive partner in the reclamation of his or her health. Responsibility will be recognized and accepted for behaviors and thought patterns that are detrimental to health and wellness. Life will be respected, and the Divine Mystery will be acknowledged. Life at all stages from the unborn to the aged will be treated with dignity. Suffering and death will be accepted as part of our life journeys, not to be feared but rather overcome through the practice of disciplines that allow wisdom, insight, and compassion.

What a joy it will be to enter again as a physician into a spiritual partnership with my patients without ingenuous attempts at rejuvenation. To address the spiritual needs of patients while realizing the mysterious interactions with our minds and bodies will be enlightening for both physician and patient. Let truth reign again in the halls of medicine.

Epilogue: Practicing Wellness

The greatest sight is to see a brave man engaged in a fight with adversity.

Seneca

The harvest is plentiful but the laborers are few.

Jesus of Nazareth

It is now time to return to my patients in the ER. They have been evaluated appropriately based on Western medical practices, and no organic crises have been identified. Now I am armed with vital healing recommendations and therapies for patients. Let us visit them again.

Robert M.

I inform Robert and his wife that all of his cardiac and pulmonary tests are normal. To a very high degree of probability there does not appear to be any heart disease present. We talk about the stressors of his home and work life, and he admits that he worries about his job constantly. He agrees that it is likely that this is the root cause of his chest pain.

I teach Robert and his wife about the importance of managing one's thought life, to rebalance one's priorities and redefine the worldly perception of success. He realizes that he has been chasing material goods and status and realizes that he may be happier in a less-lucrative job that is less stressful. We talk about meditation techniques and ways in which he can better serve his wife and family.

I tell him about these energies of stress and anxiety likely manifesting as cardiac pain in the heart chakra. He has continually felt himself distanced from his wife and family as his professional responsibilities have grown, and so his relational closeness has suffered. His heart chakra manifests these energies. I recommend several acupuncture sessions to rebalance the blockages in his heart meridian and heart chakra. I also emphasize the importance of maintaining proper exercise and diet. He is given the name of a local nutrition expert and a yoga class in his neighborhood.

Julie S.

The social worker has talked to Julie about her attachments to her depression and her life situation and the problems this is causing her. Julie admits that she is scared that she will be like this her whole life. The illusion of her belief systems is revealed, and Julie realizes that she has the potential to change and direct her own life. She acknowledges that her belief systems have been shaped by a critical, overbearing parent, and she realizes that she does not have to accept this vision of herself. Julie is given some meditation techniques and will volunteer at a local soup kitchen. She will focus on changing her attachment to her identification with herself in this condition. An appointment is made with a local psychotherapist to focus on mindfulness training.

Alice T.

The nurse is able to contact the patient's daughter. I speak with her regarding her mother's condition and modern medicine's inability to offer further quality to her life. The daughter admits to feeling tremendous guilt over a sense of abandoning her mother when she moved to the West Coast. The daughter rescinds the request for full resuscitation and requests a palliative care assessment for end-of-life care so that her mother can have some dignity as her body fails her. I assure her that her mother will not suffer as we allow her life to end in a respectful manner.

Mike R.

Mike and I talk about the numerous treatment options for lower-back pain. He is willing to try yoga and acupuncture to help his pain and alleviate his dependency on narcotics. He will see a chiropractor to help increase his mobility in his lower back. He admits that he needs to begin some light exercise and to eat healthier food. He is instructed to begin a walking regimen daily. We discuss his reliance on cigarettes and narcotics to help his pain and that these are false dependencies. Instead of focusing on his pain, Roger is instructed to focus on his pain-free periods. He is instructed to experience the pain but learn to be detached from it, to not define himself through his pain.

While in the ER I perform acupuncture on his back and legs to increase energy flow, and he feels some improvement. We schedule him an appointment with a yoga class and further mindfulness training. He promises to look into volunteer activities in the community and to become more involved in his children's lives.

Brenda F.

Brenda and her children have not been found to have evidence of a bacterial illness. We discuss the course of viral illnesses and the importance of proper eating and exercise to maintain proper health. The side effects of cough and cold remedies are discussed, and Brenda decides to use some herbal therapies for her and her children's symptoms.

Brenda realizes that her cigarette use is a coping mechanism for her stress and loneliness and has been instructed in meditation, especially her breathing. When she feels a craving for cigarettes, she will practice her breathing and awareness to realize these false dependencies. Instruction is given on the dangers of frequent antibiotic use and the need for the initiation of healthful living practices.

Melissa H.

I talk with Melissa privately and tell her that fibromyalgia is a dysfunction of imbalanced energies. Through a variety of long-term stressors, her body has retained these energies in a variety of places and can be realigned through a combination of acupuncture, chiropractic, and massage therapies.

The recent departure of her last child has been a stressor that flared up this current exacerbation. Through meditation and psychotherapy it is thought that Melissa can learn to balance her emotional stressors more effectively. Her ex-husband reenters the room at the end of our discussion and feels that these therapies will be of little benefit to his ex-wife, but does not dissuade her from trying them.

Frank L.

After a period of observation Frank exhibits no persistent adverse effects from his overdose. He feels overwhelmingly bored with himself and his life. We talk about the illusions his ego has constructed for him. He is empowered to take control of his life and promises to recommit himself to school. He would like to volunteer in a community homeless shelter. I have recommended some regular Tai Chi exercises so that he can maintain a high energy level and not be tempted to seek these energies through drug use.

Lisa G.

I tell Lisa that acupuncture would be an excellent modality to treat her migraines. She is scheduled to see an acupuncturist as an outpatient. In the meantime I show her several acupressure points to massage at the onset of future headaches. She is instructed in breathing and meditation techniques to help with her fatigue and stress. A massage therapy referral is given to help relieve her areas of manifested stress.

Henry S.

As expected, Henry's diagnostic evaluation is normal. We talk at length about the inability of Western medicine to find a causative factor for his recurrent pain. He is very open to accepting an Eastern approach to his treatment. He freely admits to being very lonely after his wife's death. He also harbors significant anger at his wife over years of marital dysfunction. Subsequently, since her death, he has been feeling significant guilt over these feelings. I recommend a session of Emotional Release Therapy for Henry and several psychotherapy sessions.

While in the ER a nurse trained in Reiki is able to administer therapy to his solar plexus and second chakra areas with significant relief of pain. It is hoped that he will be able to continue to forgive himself and his wife and release these negative energies from his solar plexus. I have also recommended a daily regimen of Qi Gong exercises to rebalance and maintain his body's energies.

My patients in the ER now had treatment options. By establishing the absence of any crisis in organ function my patients were reassured. Treatment options were offered. Detrimental behaviors were identified and accepted by the patients. There was an acceptance of the reality of the mind and spirit contributing to bodily symptoms. No medications were prescribed, so harmful side effects were avoided. After discussing test results with patients they accepted the impossibility of diagnostic certainty, yet were comforted by knowing that the test results were normal. They became aware of the mysterious mind, body, and spirit interactions and the potential for true healing.

There is an acknowledgment by physicians that scientific inquiry may not expose the causes of many ailments. Our culture, having embraced centuries of scientific progress, now turns inward to face the realities of existence. There is a cultural recognition of the inanity of most modern entertainments and a return to a focus on the brotherhood of all peoples. Destructive environmental practices are abandoned so that a purification of our food and water resources can return. The temporal nature of our physical existence is overcome by the reality of the spiritual world that is within and without. There is a profound shift of consciousness from the superficial wants and desires of the individual to the greater needs and sufferings of others. Perhaps this will be the age that sees the return of the Kingdom of Heaven.

As I finish these ramblings my thoughts return to several sights I saw this past summer as the ideas for this tome were being formulated. My home is near an airport, so I frequently witness the sights and sounds of aircraft ascending and descending. On three separate occasions as I looked skyward there was, juxtaposed in front of a climbing jet plane, a red-tailed hawk gliding in the hot summer air currents. Effortlessly maneuvering, his flight pattern was graceful, filled with a simple beauty, filled with mystery and meaning, a sharp contrast to the speeding jet aircraft in the distance. Power, speed, and efficiency contrasted against grace, beauty, and mystery.

Let us not forget in our age of technology, distraction, and stress that perhaps we are missing the obvious, ubiquitous signs of peace and grace in our busy world. Amidst mankind's desperate quest to escape the clutches of a greater truth we have lost sight of our true destinies. Perhaps we are meant to soar in the mysteries of our own beings, at peace with God and nature, awash in the bright light of grace between heaven and earth.

Maranatha

Sources

Scripture

Those seeking healing need to immerse their thought lives in scripture, the eternal sources of wisdom. I feel that the following texts represent the core readings for spiritual insight. One will find one or two texts that will become part of a daily meditation. The relative importance of the individual texts will wax and wane as your spiritual life dictates. Be open to all of these sources. The Christian will have initial difficulty accepting the wisdom of non-Christian material. Truth is Truth. One cannot turn away when confronted with eternal wisdom.

The age of fundamental, literal scripture interpretation is past. Modern scholarship has revealed that scripture has been altered through the ages by any number of scribes and interpreters. The essential truths remain, but one must proceed with caution when literal interpretation is quoted. It is imperative for the reader to know the context in which the teacher is quoted. This is all too often overlooked in textual commentary. Many religious sects criticize other traditions without ever exposing themselves to other traditions' scripture. This ignorance must cease. Realize the beauty that the world's religions reveal and learn to respect the cultures they have nourished.

The Gospel of Mark
The Bhagavad Gita
The Dhammapada
The Tao Te Ching

The Koran
The Gospel of Thomas
The Gospel of John
The Gospel of Matthew
The Gospel of Luke
Pauline Epistles
The Book of Job
Psalms
Proverbs
Upanishads
The Philokalia

Resources for Energy Work

An understanding of human energy fields is essential for growth and health maintenance. However, it is very difficult for a mind grounded in dualism and materialism to accept these realities, e.g., the Western mind. Therefore, I strongly recommend reading an overview of these systems in some detail prior to beginning a regimen of energy work.

It would be ideal to learn energy work from a teacher who is well versed in sacred and traditional energy practices. I have been fortunate to learn Qi Gong and acupuncture practices from such teachers. However, in our time the writings of these gifted instructors most typically are their only available resource. The following books have provided such a foundation for me.

Keith Sherwood, *The Art of Spiritual Healing*
J. V. Cerney, *Acupuncture Without Needles*
Yoshiaki Omura, *Acupuncture Medicine: Its Historical and Clinical Background*
Timothy McCall, MD, *Yoga as Medicine*
Walter Weston, *Pray Well: A Holistic Guide to Health and Renewal, Emotional Release Therapy*
Genevieve Lewis Paulson, *Kundalini and the Chakras*
John Mumford, *A Chakra and Kundalini Workbook*
Barbara Ann Brennan, *Hands of Light, Light Emerging*

Brugh Joy, MD, *Joy's Way, Avalanche*

Readings for Foundational Spiritual Growth and Healing

As you pursue this inner quest you will be led to writers and thinkers who will challenge your assumptions and help your spiritual growth. The following list includes many writers who have influenced my thought. It is not a finite, exclusive list; I continue to seek out other perspectives, both current and ancient. Again, truth and wisdom are not the exclusive claim of any one sect, writer, culture, or nation.

Thomas Kempis, *The Imitation of Christ*
St. Teresa of Avila, *The Interior Castle*
Meister Eckhart, *The Essential Sermons*
St. Augustine, *Confessions, The City of God*
C. S. Lewis, *Mere Christianity, The Screwtape Letters, The Problem of Pain,* and others
Philip Yancey, *Disappointment with God, Where Is God When It Hurts,* and others
Annie Dillard, *For the Time Being, Pilgrim at Tinker Creek,* and others
Richard Smoley, *Inner Christianity*
Leo Tolstoy, *Confession*
C. G. Jung, *Memories, Dreams, Reflections, Collected Works*
Thomas Merton, *No Man Is an Island, Conjectures of a Guilty Bystander,* and others
Joel S. Goldsmith, *The Art of Spiritual Healing*
Ralph Martin, *The Fulfillment of All Desire*
Wayne Meeks, *Christ Is the Question*
Dallas Willard, *The Divine Conspiracy, Renovation of the Heart*
Andrew Harvey, *The Son of Man*
Brian McLaren, *The Secret Message of Jesus*
Henri Nouwen, *Life of the Beloved, Return of the Prodigal Son*
Lee Strobel, *The Case for Faith, The Case for Christ*
John Ortberg, *The Life You've Always Wanted*
John Stott, *Life in Christ*
M. Scott Peck, *The Road Less Traveled, People of the Lie,* and others
Yoganandi, *Autobiography of a Yogi, Man's Eternal Quest*

Ernest Becker, *The Denial of Death*
Soren Kierkegaard, *Anxiety unto Death*
Andrew Weil, *Health and Healing, The Natural Mind*
Thich Nhat Hanh, *Living Buddha, Living Christ,* and others
Dietrich Bonhoeffer, *Letters and Papers from Prison, The Cost of Discipleship*
William Blake, *Poems*
John Polkinghorne, *Theology and Religion*
G. K. Chesterton, *Orthodoxy*
Wayne Meeks, ed., *The Writings of St. Paul*

Literature

Great literature reveals the human condition and augments our experience of living. The layers of illusion that coat our daily life are peeled back to reveal our real selves. The constructs of society and individuals are examined to seek truths amidst the chaos of daily living. This list is limited to books that have led me to personal spiritual insights, and I regard them as timeless in their insights.

William Shakespeare, *Hamlet, King Lear, Othello, Macbeth, The Tempest, A Midsummer Night's Dream, Much Ado About Nothing,* the sonnets
Miguel de Cervantes, *Don Quixote*
Dante Alighieri, *The Divine Comedy*
Samuel Beckett, *Waiting for Godot*
Luigi Pirandello, *Six Characters in Search of an Author*
Charles Chadwick, *It's All Right Now*
Nathaniel Hawthorne, *The Scarlet Letter*
Herman Melville, *Moby Dick*
Ralph Waldo Emerson, *Essays and Poems*
Walker Percy, *Lost in the Cosmos, Love in the Ruins, The Second Coming, The Moviegoer*
T. S. Eliot, *The Four Quartets*
Mark Twain, *Huckleberry Finn*
Ernest Hemingway, *The Sun Also Rises,* short stories
Walt Whitman, *Leaves of Grass*
Willa Cather, *My Antonia, Short Stories, Death Comes for the Archbishop*
F. Scott Fitzgerald, *The Great Gatsby, Tender Is the Night*
Gustave Flaubert, *Madame Bovary*

Jorge Luis Borges, *Ficciones*
Leo Tolstoy, *Anna Karenina, War and Peace*
Fyodor Dostoevsky, *The Brothers Karamozov, Crime and Punishment, The Idiot*
Charles Dickens, *A Christmas Carol*
J. D. Salinger, *Catcher in the Rye, Nine Stories, Franny and Zooey*
Joseph Conrad, *Heart of Darkness, Lord Jim*
John Irving, *A Prayer for Owen Meany, The Cider House Rules*
Wallace Stegner, *Angle of Repose*
Alexander Dumas, *The Count of Monte Cristo*
William Styron, *Sophie's Choice, The Confessions of Nat Turner*
Anne Tyler, *Saint Maybe*
William Faulkner, *As I Lay Dying, Light in August*
Virginia Wolff, *To the Lighthouse*
David Foster Wallace, *Infinite Jest*
Leonard Cohen, *Book of Longing*
Marianne Robinson, *Gilead*